Walks from the

G000152630

Guildford to Portsmouth

Cover photographs:

Front: *St Hubert's Church, Idsworth and the railway*

Back, LH column: *Guildford Cathedral; Cross at Gibbet Hill, Hindhead; Memorial stone to Edward Thomas at Steep; the Spinnaker Tower, Portsmouth*

Back, RH column: *River Wey near Guildford; Memorial stone bench to Octavia Hill at Hydon's Ball, Hambledon; scene on Weavers Down near Liphook; view across to Langstone from Hayling Island*

Dedicated to the memory of Andrea
May 1958 – October 2008
one of the team of friends
who helped to tread these paths.

Walks from the Railway

Guildford to Portsmouth

❧ ❧ ❧

John Owen Smith

Walks from the Railway – Guildford to Portsmouth
First published 2008

Typeset and published by John Owen Smith
19 Kay Crescent, Headley Down, Hampshire GU35 8AH

Tel: 01428 712892
wordsmith@johnowensmith.co.uk
www.johnowensmith.co.uk

ISBN 978-1-873855-55-3

Printed and bound by CPI Antony Rowe, Eastbourne

Introduction

It is about 60 miles (or 95km) to walk from Guildford to Portsmouth Harbour, and it can be done. If, however, you would prefer to let the train take at least part of the strain, this book has divided the journey into manageable chunks which can be walked between railway stations. It also includes a circular walk or two from each of the stations on the way – and I couldn't resist the temptation to offer you a quick trip to the Isle of Wight too.

The routes are described travelling towards the coast. There is no reason, of course, why you should not choose to walk in the opposite direction. In either case, I recommend that you take the relevant Ordnance Survey maps with you as, from personal experience, it can sometimes be all too easy to find yourself on the wrong path and needing to find your way back to some identifiable point. This is particularly true where a route uses permissive paths rather than public rights of way, as the former are not always shown as tracks on maps.

As usual I must thank the gallant group of friends and family who tramped these paths with me and who delighted and despaired in turn as we found unexpected gems or lost our way inexplicably when map and path mysteriously disagreed with each other.

I hope you enjoy the walks as much as we did. If you have any comments, adverse or admiring, please let me know.

John Owen Smith
September 2008

Notes:

All of the walks will have muddy patches, some will have very muddy patches – waterproof footwear is recommended in all seasons.

Where we use permissive paths rather than public rights of way, these may not always be clearly marked on the Ordnance Survey maps.

General plan of the Walks

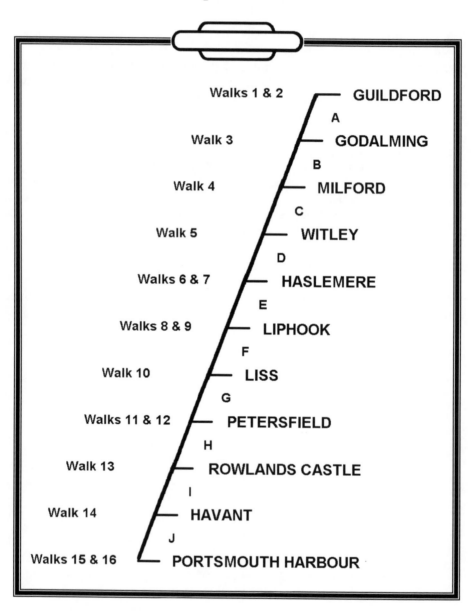

Walks 1 & 2 — GUILDFORD

A

Walk 3 — GODALMING

B

Walk 4 — MILFORD

C

Walk 5 — WITLEY

D

Walks 6 & 7 — HASLEMERE

E

Walks 8 & 9 — LIPHOOK

F

Walk 10 — LISS

G

Walks 11 & 12 — PETERSFIELD

H

Walk 13 — ROWLANDS CASTLE

I

Walk 14 — HAVANT

J

Walks 15 & 16 — PORTSMOUTH HARBOUR

The Walks

Circular Walk 1 – Guildford & Compton – 7¾ miles/12.5km 9

Circular Walk 2 – Guildford & Chilworth – 10 miles/16km 13

Link Walk A – Guildford to Godalming – 5½ miles/8.5km 16

Circular Walk 3 – Godalming & Peper Harow – 5 miles/8km 17

Link Walk B – Godalming to Milford & Witley stations –
3 miles/5km to Milford Stn; 6¾ miles/11km to Witley Stn 20

Circular Walk 4 – Milford station & Hydon's Ball – 7 miles/11km 21

Link Walk C – Between Walks 4 and 5 – ½ mile 25

Circular Walk 5 – Witley station & Chiddingfold – 8 miles/12.5km 26

Link Walk D – Witley station to Haslemere – 8½ miles/13.5km 29

Circular Walk 6 – Haslemere & Hindhead – 6 miles/9.5km 31

Circular Walk 7 – Haslemere & Blackdown – 8 miles/13km 35

Link Walk E – Haslemere to Liphook – 5½ miles/8.5km 39

Circular Walk 8 – Liphook & Bramshott – 8 miles/13km 41

Circular Walk 9 – Liphook & Griggs Green – 7½ miles/12km 47

Link Walk F – Liphook to Liss – 6 miles/9.5km 50

Circular Walk 10 – Liss & Hawkley – 9 miles/14.5km 51

Link Walk G – Liss to Petersfield – 4½ miles/7km 55

Circular Walk 11 – Petersfield & Steep – 6 miles/9.5km 57

Circular Walk 12 – Petersfield, Butser & Buriton – 11 miles/17.5km ... 61

Link Walk H – Petersfield to Rowlands Castle – 7 miles/11km 65

Circular Walk 13 – Rowlands Castle & West Marden – 8¾ miles/14km 67

Link Walk I – Rowlands Castle to Havant – 3¾ miles/6km 70

Circular Walk 14 – Havant & Hayling Island – 8½ miles/13.5km 73

Link Walk J – Havant to Portsmouth Harbour – 14 miles/22.5km 76

Circular Walk 15 – Portsmouth Harbour & Southsea – 3 miles/5km 77
Extension on the Isle of Wight: Ryde to Fishbourne – 3 miles/5km....... 79

Circular Walk 16 – Portsmouth Harbour & Gosport – 5 miles/8km 80

Other Walks and References 84

Ordnance Survey Explorer Maps covering the walks:—
>   Map 145 covers Walks 1, 2, 3 and north half of 4
>   Map 133 covers south half of Walk 4, Walks 5–11 & north half of 12
>   Map 120 covers south half of Walk 12 and Walks 13 & 14
>   Map OL29 (Isle of Wight) covers Walks 15 & 16

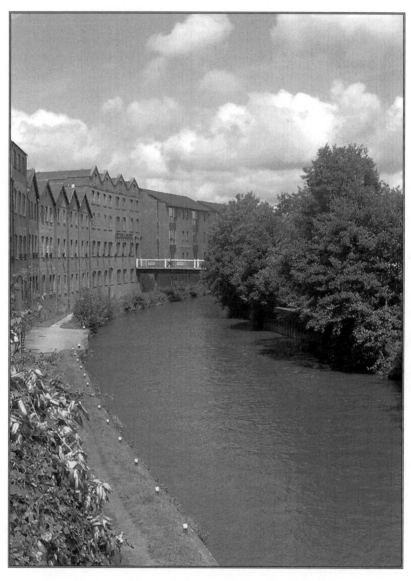

Start point: The River Wey at Guildford

Circular Walk 1 – Guildford & Compton

**Visiting: The River Wey, the North Downs Way, Compton,
the Watts Cemetery Chapel & Gallery and the end of the Hog's Back**
Distance approximately 7¾ miles/12.5km

The walk starts and ends at Guildford Station;
refreshment at *The Harrow*, Compton.

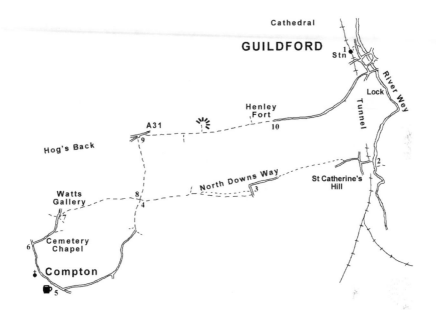

1 From the down line entrance of the station (nearest the town) turn left, then shortly turn right down steps to the River Wey (next to a pedestrian bridge over the river). Turn right (upstream) and follow the towpath. Pass under a road bridge. Note a metal sculpture of a boatman throwing a rope from a wharf on the other side of the river. Just after crossing the pedestrianised approach to another bridge into town, turn left in front of the *White House* pub to return to the riverside. Note the sculpture of Alice, her sister and the White Rabbit on the grass, celebrating Guildford's connection with Lewis Carroll. Cross a metal footbridge to arrive at Millmead Lock. The river is navigable up to Godalming. Keep following the river path upstream for another three-quarters of a mile.

2 Just before another footbridge over the river, take a path to the right sign-posted North Downs Way. This goes up Ferry Lane to cross the railway line at a point between two tunnels. St Catherine's Hill is to your left. At a road junction, turn right then left along Sandy Lane opposite *Ye Olde Ship Inn*. In a couple of hundred yards, turn right along a bridle path following the North Downs Way. Continue along this as it rises gently uphill with the Hog's Back ridge to your right.

9

3 After passing through Piccard's Farm, the track (here a farm road) turns sharp left. Here you have an option: either take the footpath on the right to continue along the North Downs Way, or take the bridleway later on the right to go along the route of the Pilgrims' Way – the latter is more shady on a hot day. The routes join in about half a mile, and the going can be very sandy underfoot in places.

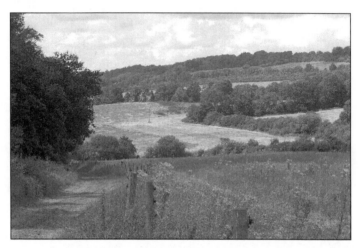

Going west along the North Downs Way

4 At a crossing of tracks (you will revisit this on your return journey, see Point 8 below), turn left down a sunken lane (which can get overgrown in summer) eventually arriving at a road (Polsted Lane) which you follow into Compton village. Turn right along the road through the village to *The Harrow* pub.

5 From the pub, continue along the road through the village, passing St Nicholas church (worth a visit) on your left.

The Pilgrims' Way is the historic route supposed to have been taken by pilgrims travelling from Winchester to the shrine of Thomas Becket at Canterbury.

St Nicholas Church, Compton contains one of the oldest surviving carved Norman screens in the country.

Watts Gallery was first opened to the public on 1 April 1904. Devoted to the art of G F Watts, it is an early example of an Arts & Crafts building and one of the first to be built in solid concrete.

The Cemetery Chapel, also completed in 1904, was designed by Mary Watts. She encouraged all from the village of Compton, whatever their social status, to learn how to model clay and make tiles to decorate the Chapel.

---

6   At the end of the village, turn right along Down Lane signposted to Watts Gallery. Take care here as there is no pavement. On your right shortly is the Watts Cemetery Chapel (open to visitors) designed by Mary Watts and further along the lane is the Watts Gallery itself, which came second in the national final of BBC's Restoration Village in 2006.

7   Turn right by the Watts Gallery along the North Downs Way. Follow this to the crossing of tracks again (Point 4 above).

8   You may of course return to Guildford from here using the route by which you came – but for an alternative with views over Guildford from high ground, turn left and follow the path which soon rises steeply to meet a road. There are views back to Compton from here.

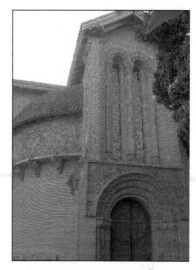

Watts Cemetery Chapel

9   Turn right, pass the gates to Compton Heights estate near to the A31 Hog's Back main road, and turn right through a metal barrier and along a wide track following the ridgeway into Guildford. The track is lined with woodland which prevents you from seeing views on either side of the ridge unless you go through it – in particular, there are good views over the cathedral from open land to the left of the track.

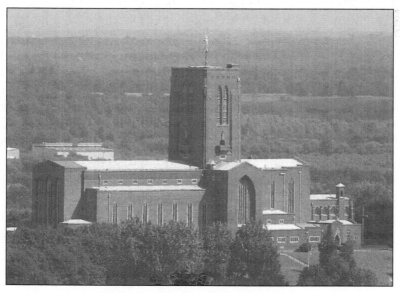

Guildford Cathedral from the ridgeway

10 Past the Henley Fort Outdoor Education Centre the track becomes a surfaced road. Keep following this downhill towards the centre of Guildford, turning left eventually to return to the railway station.

Guildford was made a diocese in 1927 and the foundation stone of the Cathedral was laid in 1936, but its building was interrupted by the Second World War. It was finally consecrated on 17th May 1961.

Henley Fort was the most westerly in a 17 mile chain of 19th century earthworks known as the London Defence Positions which would have formed a secondary line of defence if the French passed the defences on the South coast.

The London to Portsmouth shutter telegraph chain was replaced by a chain of semaphore stations which was operational from 1822 to 1847. The semaphore tower on Pewley Hill was one of these.

The River Wey was made navigable from Weybridge to Guildford by an Act of 1651, with work completed in 1653. In 1760, another Act authorised taking navigation further upstream to Godalming. Work on this was completed in 1764

The Wey and Arun Canal ran through 26 locks from the River Wey at Shalford to the River Arun at Pallingham. It was officially abandoned in 1871. Since 1970, active restoration has resulted in several miles of the waterway being restored to navigable standard. Work is continuing, with the ultimate aim of re-opening the entire canal to navigation.

Chilworth Gunpowder works was established in 1625 by the East India Company and finally closed in 1920. It was an important supplier of gunpowder to the Government. A significant number of buildings from the works can still be found – see the interpretation board at the site for details.

Circular Walk 2 – Guildford & Chilworth

Visiting: The River Wey, The Wey & Arun Canal, Chinthurst, Blackheath, Chilworth, St Martha's Church and Pewley Down
Distance approximately 10 miles/16km

The walk starts and ends at Guildford Station; refreshment at Blackheath or Guildford town centre.

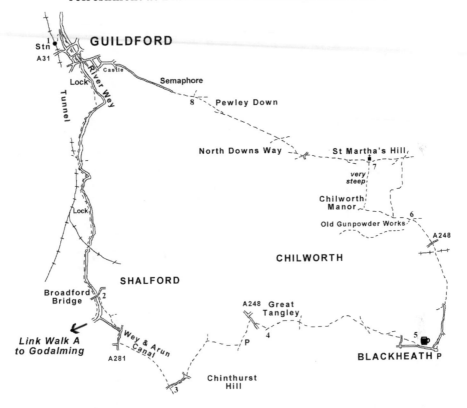

1   From the down line entrance of the station (nearest the town) turn left, then shortly turn right down steps to the River Wey (next to a pedestrian bridge over the river). Turn right (upstream) and follow the towpath. Pass under a road bridge. Note a metal sculpture of a boatman throwing a rope from a wharf on the other side of the river. Just after crossing the pedestrianised approach to another bridge into town, turn left in front of the *White House* pub to return to the riverside. Note the sculpture of Alice, her sister and the White Rabbit on the grass, celebrating Guildford's connection with Lewis Carroll. Cross a metal footbridge to arrive at Millmead Lock. The river is navigable up to Godalming. Keep following the river path upstream, past St Catherine's lock to Broadford Bridge.

If you are proceeding to Godalming (Walk A), cross the road with care and carry on straight ahead along this same bank of the river.

13

2 To continue with circular Walk 2, cross the bridge, then the road, and take the path past new industrial buildings along the other bank. It passes an old gunpowder wharf (more about that later) then diverges from the river. Just past a house on the right, bear right along a footpath by a brick pillar to arrive at a main road. There is a crossing island a few yards to the right – use this and follow the Downs Link trail opposite along the track of an old railway line. It also follows the course of the Wey & Arun Canal, which it is hoped will be restored to navigation some day.

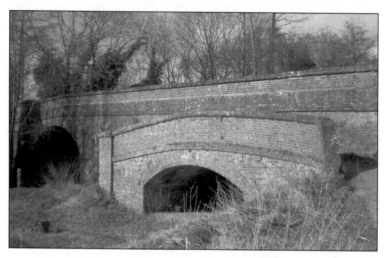

Canal bridge and Railway bridge

3 After passing under an impressive old brick railway bridge, turn left across a canal bridge (see above) overlooking the dry course of the canal. Turn left, still following the Downs Link, going up a short piece of road before taking a bridle path straight ahead at the road T-junction. The path can be muddy as it rises to a stile – from here there is a view across the Tillingbourne valley to St Martha's Church on its hill. You are heading for it, but by a more devious route. Turn right in front of the stile to continue along the Downs Link. Go past a car park (for Chinthurst Hill and its folly, up a track to the right) then cross another main road, taking the track opposite which cuts diagonally through light woodland before joining a metalled lane serving Tangley Manor and Farm.

4 Carry straight on, following the Downs Link uphill. About 250 yards after crossing a track, look for a narrow, sunken bridleway forking right by a blue-topped post and take this. Cross a road and take the bridleway opposite through light woodland, coming out by *The Villagers*. This is a walkers' pub and can be recommended for a stop.

5 From the pub, turn left and follow the road to its end in a car park. Take the bridleway halfway down the car park to the left. Follow this through woodland to where it joins a surfaced lane and stay on the lane as it passes houses

and drops downhill to a left-hand bend. Turn right along a narrow path between fences (the Downs Link again) which broadens out into a separated footpath and bridle path for a while. Cross a modern railway bridge, then cross a main road and follow the farm track ahead. As you cross the Tillingbourne stream, look for the old Chilworth gunpowder industry site on your left, with an interpretation board. Worth a visit if you have time.

6 To continue the walk, carry straight on and uphill to a T-junction of paths. For the more direct route from here to St Martha's Church, you <u>could</u> carry straight on, turn right before Chilworth Manor and take the old path straight up the hillside. This is VERY STEEP and not recommended unless you relish a long and arduous scramble (though there is a welcome seat halfway up!) For an easier climb, turn right following the Downs Link sign to meet the North Downs Way at the top of the hill – then turn left to arrive at the church.

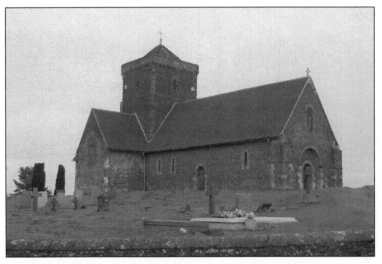

St Martha's Church on top of the hill

7 There are plenty of seats surrounding St Martha's Church, and by this time you may well feel in need of using them. To continue the walk, go west along the North Downs Way. About 50 yards after it crosses Halfpenny Lane, take a bridleway diagonally to the right. This first falls, then rises in a straight line between hedges. At a splitting of tracks, take the footpath straight ahead to reach the open space of Pewley Down at the top.

8 Follow the track to the left across the open space, taking the exit in the north-west corner into a residential road. Follow this road past the old semaphore straight down into the centre of Guildford, and find your way back to the station by one of various routes through the town shopping centre.

Link Walk A – Guildford to Godalming

Along the River Wey via Broadford Bridge and Farncombe
Distance approximately 5½ miles/8.5km

The walk starts at Guildford Station and ends at Godalming;
refreshment at Farncombe and Godalming

Follow Walk 2 to Broadford Bridge (Point 2) – then continue along the towpath down the west side of the River Wey for a further 2½ miles, passing Unstead Lock, Manor Inn (accessible from towpath), Farncombe Boat House, and Catteshall Lock to arrive in Godalming. (Note, this is not marked as a right of way on the Ordnance Survey maps).

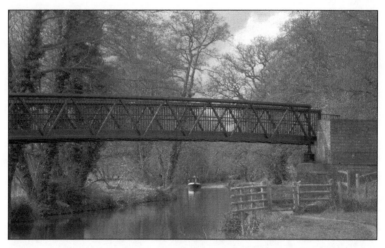

The River Wey above Broadford

Once at Town Bridge where the towpath ends, leave the river and cross the bridge – go along Bridge Street then the High Street (largely pedestrianised)

Note: To continue the walk south (see Link Walk B) turn left halfway down the High Street (at the Lloyd's Bank building) and go up Pound Lane.

Just after the 'Pepperpot' building (see photo p.19) turn right and through a gap in a wall – cross the road and take the narrow lane (Mill Lane) opposite, down hill past the *Rose & Crown* and the old mill, then uphill to the station.

Circular Walk 3 – Godalming & Peper Harow

Visiting: Westbrook, Hurtmore, Norney, Peper Harow and Eashing
Distance approximately 5 miles/8km, crossing the River Wey twice

**The walk starts and ends at Godalming Station;
refreshment at *The Squirrel*, Hurtmore or *The Stag*, Eashing.**

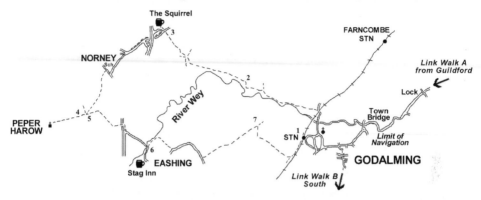

1   From the down line entrance of the station (nearest the town) follow the exit road and go along a path straight ahead where the road bears right. Turn left just in front of the church and follow the road downhill towards the River Wey. Note the Phillips Memorial Cloister and Garden on the right. Take the footbridge parallel to the road bridge over the river. Just half a mile downstream from here the river becomes navigable down to the Thames.

Godalming was the first town in Britain to have its streets lit by electricity, in September 1881 – but by 1884 the town had reverted back to gas lighting due to problems with the electricity supply.

The town hall, nicknamed the Pepperpot, dates back to 1814 and has become the logo of Godalming.

Phillips Memorial Cloister was created in memory of Jack Phillips, one of the radio operators on the *Titanic*, who was born in Godalming.

Go through a car park before rejoining the road to pass under the railway. Take a footpath to the left just before another bridge over a stream, and follow this stream past Westbrook Mill and onwards until it runs beside the river through Access Land. Where paths diverge, keep to the path by the river, finally taking an uphill path by a WW2 pillbox to the end of a residential road.

2 Turn left along a footpath signposted to Shackleford which clings to the slope of the river valley. Follow this past a building with gardens on the left, then go straight ahead at a crossroads of paths and uphill along a surfaced track to pass below a road and arrive at *The Squirrel Inn*, recommended for a refreshment stop.

3 Going out of the *Squirrel Inn* car park, cross the road and turn left, then turn right along a pavement by the roadside to pass under the A3. Where the road forks, take the left lane towards Norney. At a T-junction, turn right past the village school and shortly take a footpath on the left. This soon crosses fields to arrive at stile at a junction of tracks.

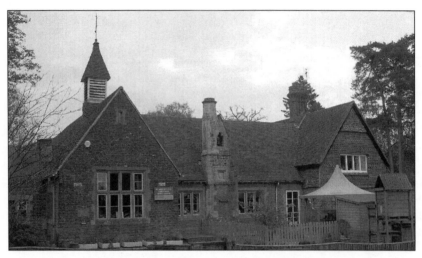

St Mary's C of E village school at Norney

4 If you wish to visit the private estate of Peper Harow with its old church and its park landscaped by 'Capability' Brown, go straight ahead through a small section of wood, then over another stile and across a field by the cricket field. Retrace your steps back to the junction of tracks to continue the walk.

5 Coming from Peper Harow, turn right at the junction and through a metal gate, then follow the bridleway round the edge of a field and over the A3 on an accommodation bridge. Turn left along the road to Eashing, crossing the River Wey again on a bridge where traffic is controlled by lights. If you wish to visit the nearby *Stag Inn* for refreshment, follow the road as it bears right and passes the site of Eashing Mill. To continue the walk, turn left at the end of the bridge along a public footpath.

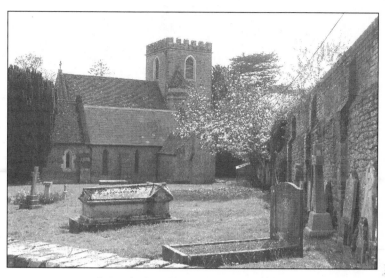

St Nicholas Church, Peper Harow

6   The path rises to a stile, then crosses a field to a road by a bungalow. Turn left along the road, proceeding with care as there is no pavement. Shortly, turn left along Halfway Lane and follow where it bends sharply right at the end.

7   The lane becomes a sunken path which descends towards the railway line in the valley. Follow it to the west entrance of Godalming Station.

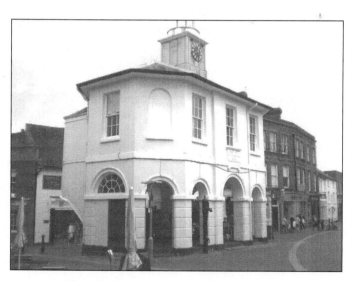

The 'Pepperpot' building in Godalming

19

Link Walk B –Godalming to Milford Stn or Witley Stn

Distance approximately 3 miles/5km to Milford Station
or 6¾ miles/11km to Witley Station
or 5½ miles/9km to Hambledon for connection to all points south

The walk starts at Godalming Station and ends at either Milford Station or Witley Station

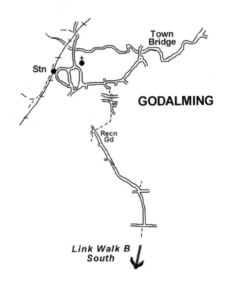

From the down line entrance of Godalming station (nearest the town) turn right and follow the exit road (Mill Lane) down past the old mill buildings, then uphill past the Rose & Crown – cross a road and go through a gap in the wall to the High Street.

Turn left along the pedestrianised High Street, forking to the right at the 'Pepperpot', and halfway along (at the Lloyd's Bank building) turn right up Pound Lane. Take the left fork, then just before the nursing home entrance take a footpath to the right between walls. Follow the path to a light-controlled crossing of the bypass.

Cross the bypass and turn right along the pavement, then shortly left at railings and up a path. Turn left at the top where it meets a road, then shortly right up Latimer Road. Take a footpath forking to the right which climbs steeply to a recreation ground at the top.

Turn right along a footpath which borders a recreation ground to meet Busbridge Lane. Turn left along this road and follow it over a crossroads and to a T-junction. Carry straight on here along a bridleway which soon descends between walls to lakes (listen for the sounds of wildfowl) where it meets another path coming from the right. This is Point 3 on **Circular Walk 4**.

*For the shortest route to Milford Station, turn right here and follow **Circular Walk 4** in the reverse direction for another 1½ miles. Alternatively carry straight on and follow it in the direction described for 5 miles.*

*For Witley Station and all points south, carry straight on and follow **Circular Walk 4** in the direction described until Point 7, then follow **Link Walk C**.*

20

Circular Walk 4 – Milford station & Hydon's Ball

Visiting: Tuesley, Busbridge Lakes, Hydon's Ball, Hambledon Church, Great Enton and part of Witley
Distance approximately 7 miles/11km

The walk starts and ends at Milford Station; refreshment at *The Merry Harriers*, Hambledon.

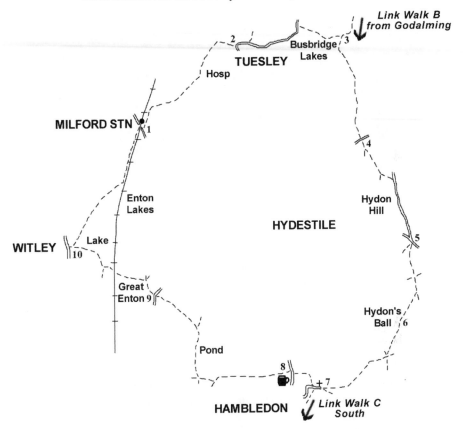

1   From Milford station, turn left and take Summer Lane following the railway track north. It soon diverges to the right, passing between a golf course and a horticultural farm. The large 'poly-tunnels' here were among the first in the country to become subject to planning laws. Carry straight on when the track becomes a path which dips to cross a stream, then rises through a sunken section to pass the rear of Milford Hospital. Cross a field by the side of the hospital to arrive at a road.

2   Turn left to follow the road downhill and for a further half a mile (taking care of traffic) until it turns sharp left. A few yards after this bend take a footpath to the right which goes along the side of a fishing lake. Sadly the pond is stoutly fenced off from the path so that views of it are restricted.

21

3 Turn right at a T-junction of tracks and cross a temporary bridge between ponds – again the view of both is unfortunately restricted. The track rises then, sunken in places, passes between a field and a wood to pass Clock Barn Farm and reach a road.

4 Cross the road and take the paved drive opposite, shortly bearing left off the drive and along a bridleway. When this meets another road, turn right, soon passing the entrance to Hydon Hill Cheshire Home to arrive at a triangular T-junction of roads.

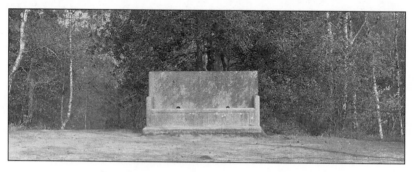

Seat on Hydon's Ball with inscription:
"This land was given in memory of Octavia Hill 1915"

5 Cross straight over with care to enter National Trust land and follow the track straight ahead used by vehicles, carrying on where this turns into a car park. Soon after crossing another track, look for an unsigned path going diagonally to the right (by a cluster of concrete SV markers) which rises to the top of Hydon's Ball. The area is dedicated to the memory of Octavia Hill (1858–1912), one of the founders of the National Trust, and there is a large inscribed stone seat at the top of the hill to mark this.

> The National Trust was founded in 1895 by Octavia Hill, Sir Robert Hunter and Canon Hardwicke Rawnsley. Sir Robert is commemorated at Waggoners Wells – see Circular Walk 8.

6 Carry straight on over the clearing at the top of the hill to descend the other side by one of several unsigned paths. At a cross-roads of tracks, take the one going downhill through an old coppice wood, and at a further cross-roads of tracks turn right at the bottom along a level path to reach a metal kissing-gate into a field. Cross the field diagonally on a clear sandy path through the crop, going through another gate and another field before arriving at Hambledon Church and its associated attractive old houses.

7 The path becomes a paved road as it goes past the church wall. *The link Walk C to Witley station and all points south bears left here along the Greensand Way.* Just as the road starts to go downhill, take a track to the right which descends and bends to meet a road by a touring caravan site at a kissing-gate opposite the *Merry Harriers* pub which, despite its boast of "Warm Beer and Lousy Food" is a good stopping point.

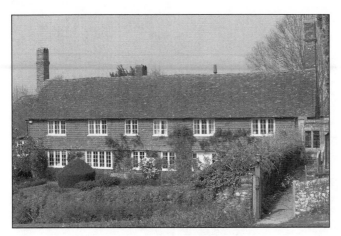

Houses next to Hambledon Church

8 Proceed along the Public Bridleway down the right hand side of the pub. After about half a mile, take a footpath to the right in light woodland. Shortly turn right again along another footpath – this leads shortly to a metal gate and through a meadow. The buildings of Enton Hall are to the left and a pond to the right. At the end of the meadow take the path straight ahead through a kissing-gate and up a slope across another field. Follow this path for about 700 yards to a road.

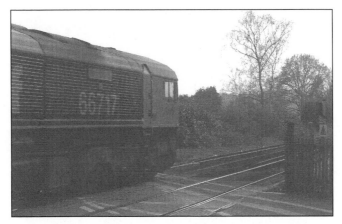

'Good Old Boy' crossing Milford level crossing

9 Cross the road and go down the service track opposite leading to Great Enton. Turn left in front of a tile-fronted house to follow the track under the railway and past the attractive Enton Mill Farm towards Witley.

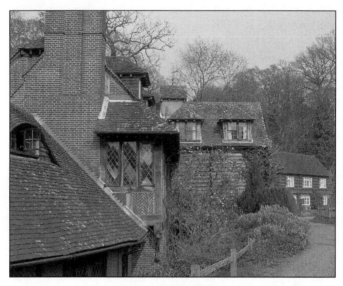

Enton Mill Farm

10 Just before reaching Witley, turn sharp right along a public footpath by the Social Club bowls green. This crosses a road and continues as a track leading to allotments, then as a narrow fenced path which eventually turns to follow the railway line embankment for a straight 600 yards back to the level crossing at Milford station.

Link Walk C – between Walks 4 and 5

Between Hambledon church and Oakhurst Cottage
Distance approximately ½ mile

From Hambledon church, take the Greensand Way south-west. This passes through a kissing-gate and across two fields before dropping to meet a road via a house drive. Turn left along the road, taking care round a blind bend where there is no footpath. Shortly, at a road junction, go slightly left down an accommodation road past terraced houses. Follow this – it becomes a narrow track, going downhill to meet another road. Cross the road and follow the marked right-of-way across the gravel in front of a house and past garages into the woods. Shortly, when it meets a more substantial track used by vehicles, turn right, then at a T-junction turn left down a narrow track leading to the National Trust property Oakhurst Cottage.

Circular Walk 5 continues from here from its Point 3. For Witley Station, turn right and follow it in the reverse direction for 1½ miles. For Chiddingfold and all points south, turn left and follow it in the direction described.

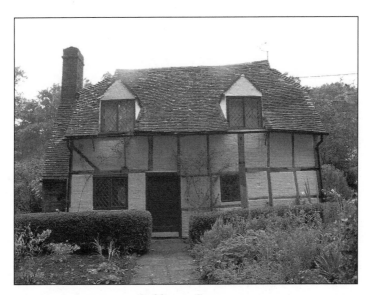

Oakhurst Cottage

Oakhurst Cottage is a small 16th Century timber-framed cottage containing furniture and artefacts reflecting several centuries of continued occupation. There is a delightful cottage garden. Visits by appointment only (40 minute guided tour). Maximum of 6 people at any one time. Open April to October. Enquiries: (01428) 684090.

Circular Walk 5 – Witley Station & Chiddingfold

Visiting: Wormley, Hambledon, Oakhurst Cottage, Hambledon Hurst, Chiddingfold, Langhurst and Sandhills
Distance approximately 8 miles/12.5km

The walk starts and ends at Witley Station; refreshment in Chiddingfold

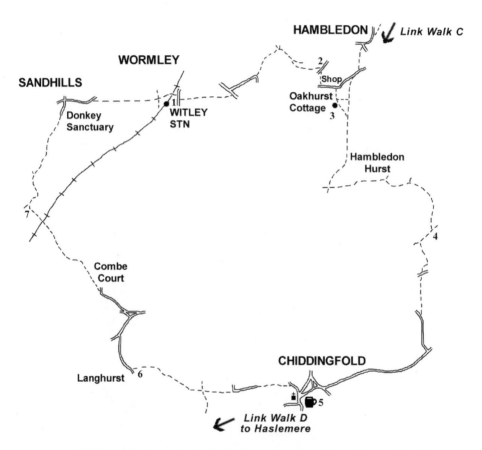

1 From Witley Station, go down the exit road, cross the main road and take the footpath through barriers opposite. This is the waymarked Greensand Way (GW). Follow this between fences to a main road. Turn left, then right along Wormley Lane, still following the GW. Where the lane bears sharp right, go straight ahead through woodland to a junction of several tracks in front of a half-timbered house. Here you follow the GW along a bridleway to the right of the house. As you come out onto heathland, near the top of a rise fork right continuing along the bridleway and diverging from the GW (although older maps show the bridleway as the GW). This takes you downhill and through woodland to a road.

2 Turn right along the road, then shortly sharp left down a track towards houses, then sharp right along a narrow surfaced footpath. This comes out at a road by Hambledon village shop. Turn left along the road with the green and its cricket square on your right, then turn right along a track signposted to Oakhurst Cottage, keeping the green on your right. Continue down this track past the point where it narrows to a footpath. On your right is Oakhurst Cottage (see details on p.25).

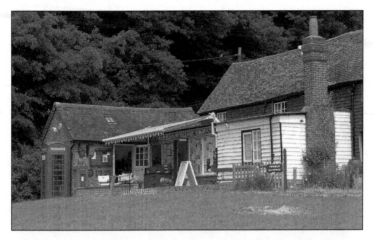

Hambledon shop, run by the village for the village

3 From Oakhurst Cottage, continue through a wooden barrier and down the track which soon merges with a public bridleway carrying on in the same direction, through woods, muddy in places. In about half a mile at a crossing of bridleways, turn sharp left. Follow this less well-defined track for about half a mile, bearing right where the rights-of-way divide. Shortly, bear right again at another junction of bridleways and follow this track through woods and finally downhill to meet a bridleway at a T-junction in a valley.

4 Turn right, and in a few yards go left over a substantial footbridge across a deep-cut stream. Follow this bridleway uphill to meet a paved drive. Cross the drive and go straight ahead along the edge of a field and past a timbered and tile-hung cottage to emerge on a road. Turn left along the road, and shortly right at a T-junction towards Chiddingfold and its large village green. In Chiddingfold, the *Crown* is said to be the oldest pub in Surrey.

> The name Chiddingfold was once synonymous with glass manufacture. The first glass-master known by name to have worked in England was Laurence Vitrearius, who arrived from Normandy and established himself at Pickhurst near Chiddingfold in 1226. His name appears in the records of Westminster Abbey in 1240 as being one of the people associated with the production of glass for the east end.

5   Cross the main road with care. *For Haslemere and all points south, turn left along the pavement then shortly right along Mill Lane to join Link Walk D in half a mile at Sydenhurst.* To continue this circular walk, turn right in front of the church and follow the pavement along the road. Round a corner, take a footpath forking to the left passing through a metal kissing gate by the churchyard. Follow the narrow strip of metalled path uphill across a field to meet the end of a residential road. Go along this, and where it turns right follow the path straight ahead between fences. Cross a double stile into a field and follow the path along its length. (Midway along this, another footpath crosses – see Link Walk D which leaves here.) Follow the path over several stiles to meet a lane (Pook Hill).

6   Turn right along the lane, passing Langhurst Manor and bearing right at a road junction. In about 150 yards, turn left down the drive to Combe Court Farm and shortly go through a metal gate on the right and follow the surfaced track to the left (signs say 'Public footpath'). At the top of a hill, take the stile over the metal fence to the left and follow the footpath. Follow this for about a mile. It descends and crosses a deep-banked stream in a wooded valley (very muddy at times) before crossing the railway line at a pedestrian level crossing (take normal precautions here) before meeting a bridleway at a T-junction.

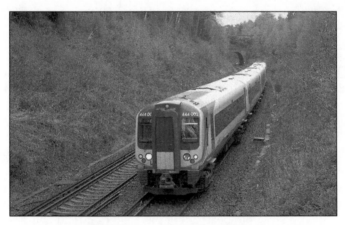

Southbound train approaching Witley station

7   Turn right and follow the bridleway across a wooden footbridge and for three-quarters of a mile to a road, passing a donkey sanctuary on the right. This area is known as Sandhills. Turn right along the road, then shortly where the road bears left carry straight on along a track waymarked Greensand Way (GW). Follow this. After it crosses the railway on a footbridge, go through a gap in the fence to the right to return to Witley Station.

Link Walk D – Witley Station to Haslemere

Visiting: Combe Court, Sydenhurst, Frillinghurst, and Imbhams
Distance approximately 8½ miles/13.5km

The walk starts at Witley Station and ends at Haslemere Station

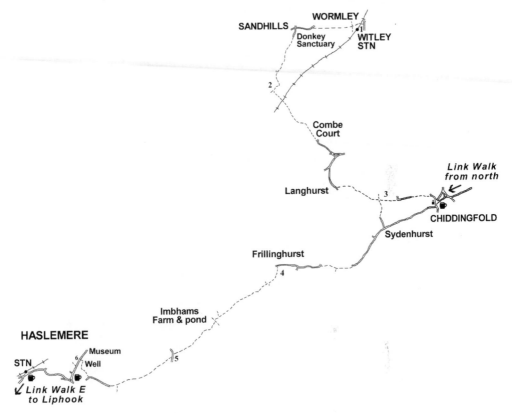

1   *Start by following Circular Walk 5 in reverse direction (see further details in previous section).* From Witley station entrance, turn left through the car park and go through a gap in the fence to a footpath. Turn left over the railway and follow this path to join a road. Follow the road to a crossroads with Hatch Lane. Turn left here. Passing a donkey sanctuary on the left, the lane becomes a bridleway, and we follow this for three-quarters of a mile.

2   Shortly after crossing a stream, turn left along a footpath which goes across the railway (take care) and a wooded valley (muddy) and across fields to join a paved track to Combe Court. Follow this downhill to meet a road. Turn right, then after about 200 yards fork left along Pook Hill. After a quarter of a mile take a footpath across a stile to the left. Follow this across fields and more stiles for about half a mile to a crossroads of footpaths (not obvious – look for a stile in the hedge on the left for a clue). *Here we leave Circular Walk 5.*

3 Turn right along the footpath leading through woods and past a pond then through a gate and along a drive to Sydenhurst on Mill Lane. Turn right along the lane, and carry straight on where it becomes a bridleway. After three-quarters of a mile it meets another lane. Turn left here, and where the lane bends left, take a farm road straight ahead to Frillinghurst. This area was the heart of a local ironworking industry up to the eighteenth century. After going through the farm buildings, cross a stile into a field on the left.

4 Cross two fields (meadows at the time of writing) following the footpath. Continue along this path for just over three-quarters of a mile through woodland and across a wooden bridge over a stream to a junction of tracks by the pond at Imbham's Farm.

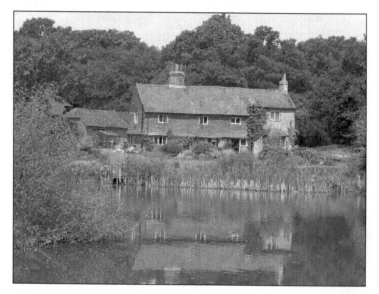

Imbham's Farm and pond

Turn left and go along the track by the side of the pond, then follow it as it bears right and after half a mile leads to a road.

5 Cross the road, taking the footpath opposite. The path crosses a number of fields, some linked with plank bridges over ditches. Circular Walk 7 and the Serpent Trail join us from the left. The path passes through a kissing gate and joins a lane – when the lane turns left, go through another kissing gate on the right and follow a footpath across a field towards buildings. Go through another gate and turn right arriving at Haslemere Town Well set in a wall (see p.38). This is the end of the Serpent Trail (see p.36). Turn left for the High Street.

6 At the High Street, turn left down the hill – refreshment may be taken at a number of places here. Turn right after the War Memorial and follow the road for another half a mile to the railway station.

Circular Walk 6 – Haslemere & Hindhead

Visiting: Inval, Hindhead Common and Gibbet Hill
Distance approximately 6 miles/9.5km

**The walk starts and ends at Haslemere Station;
refreshment at Hindhead**

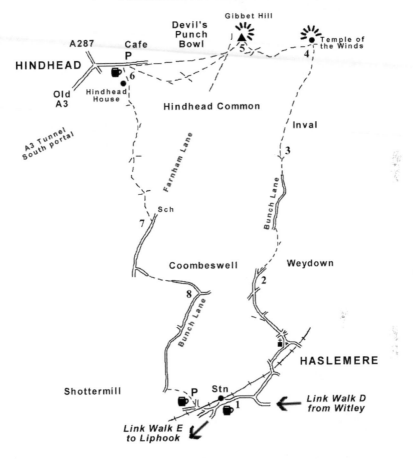

1 Turn left out of the station, and follow the road towards Haslemere. Turn left along Tanners Lane, cross the railway bridge at the end and follow the road to the right. Keep to the left as the road passes St Bartholomew's Church and follow it (High Lane) up and over a hill.

2 Take the drive forking to the right to Wispers School and soon bear left along a parallel bridle path, later taking a left fork which leads to a road (Bunch Lane). Turn right and follow this for just under half a mile to its end. The tarmac ends and it passes through a locked metal barrier.

3 Carry straight on up the central of three bridleways. This rises through trees in a fairly straight line before levelling off. After a bit more than half a mile

31

you arrive at a T-junction of tracks with a large octagonal stone base straight ahead – this is known locally as the 'Temple of the Winds' (see Circular Walk 7 for another) with views to the north.

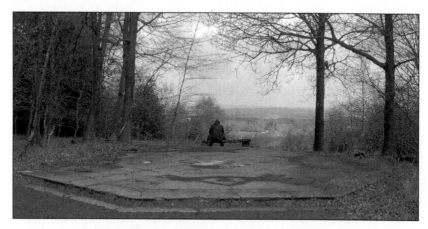

The base of the 'Temple of the Winds'

4   Turn left and follow the track for just under half a mile to a metal barrier where a BOAT (Byway Open to All Traffic) crosses. Take the path straight ahead which rises sharply to the top of Gibbet Hill – on a clear day it is possible to see London from here.

5   Turn left, heading approximately south-west from the triangulation point, over the grass to a rectangular area which once was a car park. Cross this and take the footpath ahead, ignoring the track through a metal barrier to the left. If you prefer you can take the track to the right and walk along the now-paved original coach road from London to Portsmouth past the 'Sailor's Stone' on its way to Hindhead village; the suggested path gives a more open walk across Hindhead Common parallel to the coach road. Either brings you to the old A3 opposite the National Trust car park and restaurant. Take refreshment here or at the Devil's Punch Bowl Hotel.

> After many years of deliberation, work began in 2008 to construct a twin tunnel taking the A3 London to Portsmouth road under Hindhead and away from the National Trust land at the Devil's Punch Bowl.

6   Turn left before the Hotel to take the bridleway (part of the Greensand Way) which runs through woodland down the west side of Hindhead Common behind Tyndall's Estate. Accessible through a gap in the hedge, *Hindhead House*, built in 1884 for Professor John Tyndall FRS, was the first house on Hindhead. At that time it had uninterrupted views of open heathland in all directions, but developers soon moved in and Tyndall erected 40ft-high

screens of birch and heather around his property to shield himself from his neighbours! The house remains, now converted into flats.

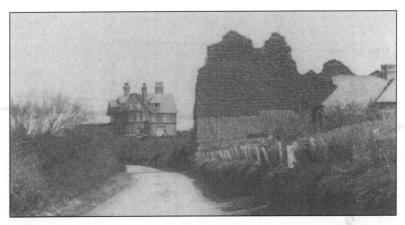

Hindhead House with one of Prof Tyndall's screens in the 1880s (taken looking up the road from Haslemere, now the A287)

Follow the bridleway downhill through a National Trust gate (which keeps grazing animals in) and across a valley with a fence and a gate on your right, then uphill through more open country with views to the right over Polecat valley. Continue to follow signs for the Greensand Way as it rises sharply (sharing a track with an embedded pipeline) and through another NT gate to arrive at a road (Farnham Lane).

7   Turn right to follow the lane downhill for a quarter of as mile, then turn left along the Greensand Way – at first a drive, then a rough 'hollow lane' to the left of Pucksfold, going steeply down to become a metalled road again. Follow this to its junction with another road (Bunch Lane again).

8   Turn right along the road, and follow it for just over half a mile. Take a footpath to the left. This brings you out beside a car park. If you need refreshment at this point, the *Crown and Cushion* pub is at hand. Follow the main road under the railway bridge to return to the station.

> Haslemere was, quite literally, on the road to nowhere until the railway arrived in 1859 and opened up the area as a commuter belt. Ready access to and from London put pressure on the surrounding common land including Hindhead, giving in-comers incentives to buy and to build. In short, the area was from then on earmarked for invasion.

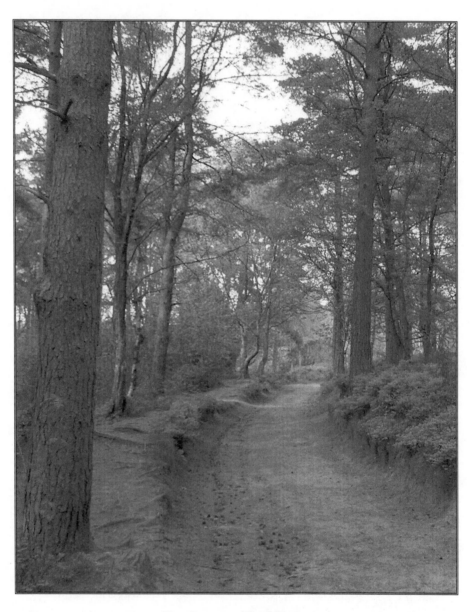

Track across Black Down

Circular Walk 7 – Haslemere & Blackdown

Visiting: Camelsdale, Marley Common, Valewood, Blackdown and Haslemere
Distance approximately 8 miles/13km

**The walk starts and ends at Haslemere Station;
refreshment in Haslemere**

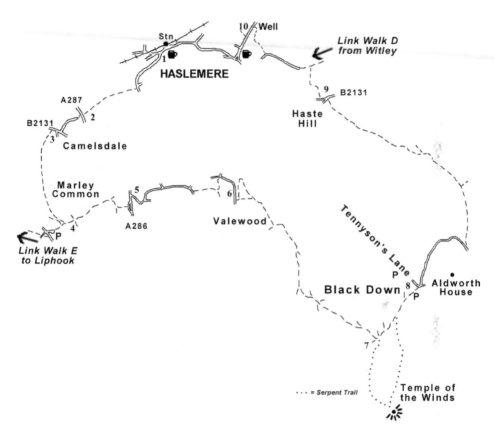

1 Turn right out of the station, cross the road at the pedestrian crossing and take Longdene Road opposite. Follow it uphill, and just after its junction with Courts Hill Road take a footpath to the right. This descends between fields to a stile then past some buildings (Sturt Farm) to a main road.

2 Cross the road with care, taking the footpath opposite down to the end of a residential road. Follow this road up to a T-junction. Turn right, then shortly left at Marley Combe Road taking the footpath immediately to the right up steps into National Trust land.

3 Follow the track rising up through woodland for nearly three-quarters of a mile. Note that the obvious path is not the public right of way marked on the OS map, which starts in a more sunken lane to the right – they begin on

35

parallel courses but diverge later. Either path will do. Continue for about three-quarters of a mile from the bottom until on Marley Common it crosses the Sussex Border Path, where you turn left. *This is where Link Walk E leaves us, taking the Sussex Border path to the right.*

4 Follow the Sussex Border Path (also waymarked at this point as the Serpent Trail,[†] which you will follow from here back to Haslemere.) It eventually descends steeply behind houses and across a drive to emerge at a main road.

5 Turn left and cross the road with care to take Fernden Lane opposite. After a bend, turn left along a bridleway. Follow signs for both The Serpent Trail and the Sussex Border Path, through a gateway at Lake House and across duckboards over marshy areas to arrive at the drive to Valewood Farm House.

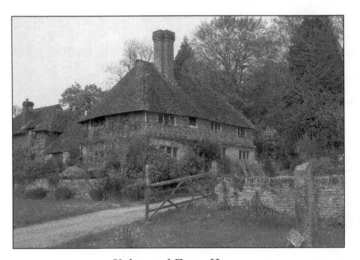

Valewood Farm House

6 Follow the drive past the house, then take a track to the left which curves further left into National Trust land (Valewood Park). After passing through a gate you have the option of a short sharp climb across the field to your right or a more leisurely stroll up the circuitous track to the top. Go through another gate, across an open field and through a further gate. Follow the signed route left. It passes through rhododendrons, then another gate leads to open woodland. Keep to the marked Serpent Trail, arriving eventually on the wooded top of Blackdown.

7 Here the Serpent Trail diverges from the Sussex Border Path – the former takes you on a mile-long diversion to visit Tennyson's favourite 'Temple of

---

[†] The Serpent Trail is a 64-mile long waymarked path which winds its way from Haslemere to Petersfield by way of Petworth and Midhurst, designed to showcase the landscape of the greensand hills in West Sussex. A Guide to the trail is published by the South Downs Joint Committee – ISBN 978-1-900543-42-2

the Winds' viewpoint; the latter misses this and proceeds directly along the main track towards the National Trust car parks on Tennyson's Lane. Fork right and downhill following a bridleway sign and through a National Trust gate to arrive on the road opposite the drive to *Aldworth*.

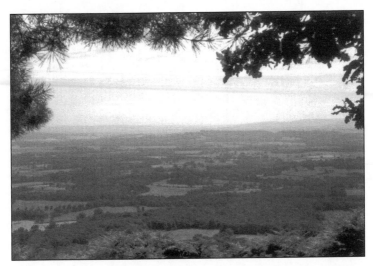

View south-east from the 'Temple of the Winds', Blackdown

Alfred Tennyson, Poet Laureate, decided in 1866 to move from the Isle of Wight to avoid the sightseers there. He found his ideal spot and moved into his new house *Aldworth* in 1869. Built of local sandstone 800 feet up on Blackdown it was a pioneering effort, only possible for a relatively wealthy person. It was equipped with all the conveniences then required by an increasingly sophisticated middle class – it even had a bath, something that his other house in the Isle of Wight lacked.

Tennyson wrote about the view from his 'Temple of the Winds':—

> *"You came, and look'd and loved the view*
> *Long-known and loved by me.*
> *Green Sussex fading into blue*
> *With one grey glimpse of sea."*

8 Follow the road past the drive to *Aldworth* and downhill. After about half a mile, at the entrance gate to Barfold, take the bridleway to the left. Follow this for just over half a mile to High Barn Farm, where the track deviates on a diversion between fences to the right. Take the path through a gate on your left in front of the house and across a field to another gate. This leads to a path through woodland which eventually joins a drive leading to a road. Note the old almshouses to the right on the opposite side.

9 Cross the road with care and turn left along the wide verge, soon taking a footpath to the right. This descends through National Trust woodland, across some plank bridges and through a couple of kissing gates to a junction of tracks.

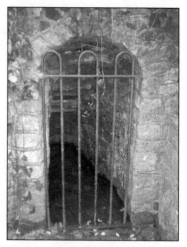

Turn left here, following the Serpent Trail. The path passes through a kissing gate and joins a lane – when the lane turns left, go through another kissing gate on the right and follow a footpath across a field towards buildings. Go through another gate and turn right arriving at Haslemere Town Well set in a wall. This is the end of the Serpent Trail. Turn left for the High Street.

10 At the High Street, turn left down the hill – refreshment may be taken at a number of places here. Turn right after the War Memorial and follow the road for another half a mile to the railway station.

Haslemere Town Well

At the High Street, turn right up the hill to visit Haslemere Educational Museum, a few doors away.

In 1888 the Quaker surgeon Sir Jonathan Hutchinson founded a museum in the grounds of his home at *Inval* in Haslemere. Determined to offer educational opportunities to local people he allowed the public to enjoy his life's collection of objects of interest in the field of botany, geology and social history. The huge popularity of the Museum led to the launch of an innovative series of lectures and activities which still continues today. In 1926 the Museum arrived at its present site with its Georgian facade in the High Street.

The museum is independent and relies on the financial support of visitors and members. Entry by donation. Closed on Sundays and Mondays.

Link Walk E – Haslemere to Liphook

Visiting: Camelsdale, Marley Common, Linchmere and Stanley Common
Distance approximately 5½ miles/8.5km

The walk starts at Haslemere Station and ends at Liphook Station

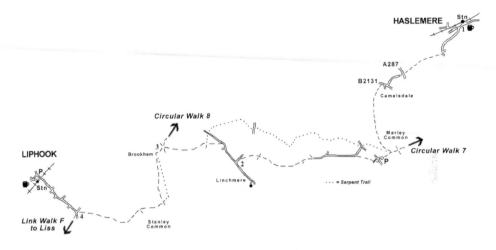

1 *Start by following* **Circular Walk 7** *from Haslemere Station to Point 4 (see details in previous section).* For Link Walk E, turn right onto the Sussex Border Path (SBP) at this point.

Note that the Serpent Trail also links Marley Common to Liphook, but uses a slightly different route at times, often over permissive paths which are not shown clearly on the Ordnance Survey maps – however it is generally well waymarked. Choose whichever you like – we describe the SBP route here.

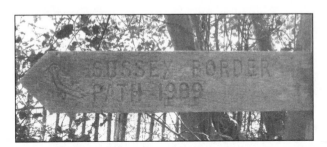

Signpost along the Sussex Border path

The SBP passes though a NT car park to a road. Cross the road taking the drive opposite, and shortly turn right where a track crosses. Follow this track (waymarked SBP) through trees, and where it emerges at a road junction take the road straight ahead past houses. Continue to follow the SBP, first along

39

the road then along a well-defined track for about 1½ miles to Linchmere (also spelt Lynchmere), joining a road at the end. Turn left towards a T-junction.

> For a fascinating visit to St Peter's Church, turn left at the T-junction. The church is just under a quarter of a mile along the road.
>
> Note in particular the carved lamb by the font inside the church, and the peaceful rural view to the south from the churchyard.
>
> Return to the junction to continue Link Walk E.

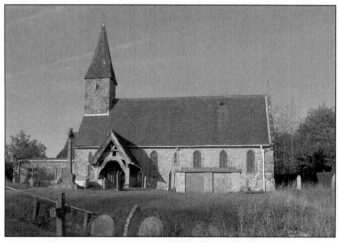

St Peter's Church, Linchmere from the south

2   Turn right at the T-junction and follow the road for about a quarter of a mile before turning left along a track (waymarked SBP) just after Danley Lane. This joins the Serpent Trail after about 200 yards, and they share much of the rest of the route. Half a mile from the road you come to a 5-way junction of tracks. *This is Point 3 on **Circular Walk 8**, which joins us here – we follow it in reverse direction to arrive at Liphook station.*

3   Follow the waymarks with care as there are several unmarked paths to divert you (I speak from experience!) – but, all being well, about a mile and a quarter after the 5-way junction you should arrive at the road to Liphook at its junction with Highfield Lane.

4   If you wish to proceed to Liss and all points south, take the track opposite Highfield Lane and follow **Link Walk F**. Otherwise follow the road into Liphook to arrive at the station.

Circular Walk 8 – Liphook & Bramshott

Visiting: Stanley Common, Hammer Vale, Bramshott Common, Waggoners Wells, Bramshott and its churchyard and Liphook centre
Distance approximately 8 miles/13km

The walk starts and ends at Liphook Station;
refreshment mid-point at the *Prince of Wales*, Hammer Vale

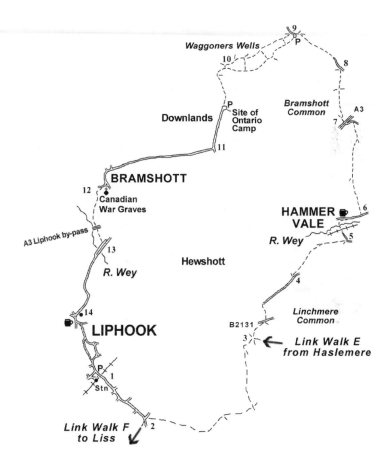

1   Turn right out of the station and into the car park. Take the steps up to the road bridge, and cross the railway line. Follow the road, crossing to use the pavements as necessary. Just past the 'Welcome to West Sussex' sign, turn left into Highfield Lane, and almost immediately take a bridleway to the right.

2   Follow the bridleway, which is the Sussex Border Path. After about a mile, when it drops into a valley, turn left at a crossroads of tracks and follow the valley downhill.

41

3   Just after passing an almost hidden house, there is a 5-way junction of tracks. *Link Walk E joins here, moving in the opposite direction.* Take the second exit to the left (a footpath) which goes across 'open access' land and soon arrives at a road. Cross the road with care (the traffic moves fast here) and up the bridleway opposite. On passing a sign for Tiggers Field, the track starts to become an accommodation road for houses. Follow the road as far as Gillham's Farm before taking the second of two bridleways through a gate to the left.

4   The track goes gently downhill through a lightly wooded section, then through a meadow before reaching a road at a gate.

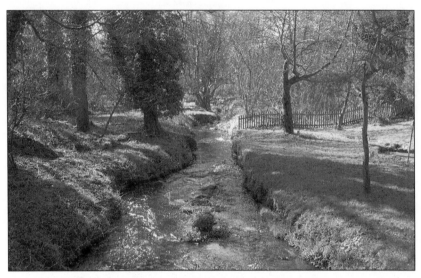

The young River Wey at Hammer Vale

5   Turn left along the road, through Hammer Farm yard and over the railway on a pedestrian level crossing (take usual care), then over a stream which is the young River Wey and up a track past houses to a road. This is the hamlet of Hammer Vale, named after the ironworks which existed near here in earlier days. Turn left here to visit the *Prince of Wales* pub, or turn right to continue the walk.

6   Shortly turn left up a footpath by the wall of a house garage. The footpath climbs through heathland. At the top, bear right to follow a wide track below electricity power lines. This eventually leads to a minor road close to its junction with the A3.

To the left of the wide track is an area which has been used during two World Wars as a military hospital. The Connaught Hospital, here during the Second World War, was finally closed in 1962.

---

7 Cross the dual carriageway A3 with care through a gap in the crash barriers. Go through an access gate on the other side to enter Bramshott Common. Descend into a valley, turning right then left to follow a footpath uphill and across the common, crossing another track to arrive at a gate leading to a grass path between house gardens. This leads to a paved road.

8 Turn left along the road which eventually becomes a water-eroded bridleway heading downhill to the ford at the head of Waggoners Wells ponds.

9 Cross the ford and take the track to the left along the side of the pond. To the right of the path is Sir Robert Hunter's stone.

Sir Robert Hunter, who lived in Haslemere, founded the National Trust with Octavia Hill (see Circular Walk 4) and Canon Rawnsley in 1895. He died in 1913, and Waggoners Wells, the first local property to be acquired by the Trust following his death, is dedicated to his memory.

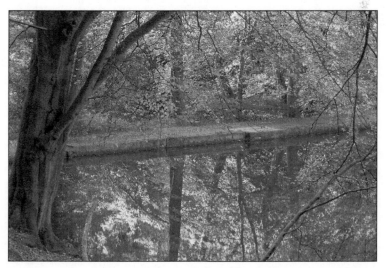

Reflections at Waggoners Wells

Three man-made ponds form the chain known as Waggoners Wells. The walk may be continued down either side of the ponds, crossing over at the dams. Note the small quarry in the north bank by each dam – it was from here that material was taken to build them, some 400 years ago. At the dam to the third (and last) pond, take the right-hand side, and follow the path passing to the left of *Summerden* down to the National Trust wishing well.

Waggoners (or Wakeners) Wells were constructed as hammer ponds in the 1630s by Henry Hooke, who already had ironworks at Hammer Vale. For some reason, however, no industry ever developed here.

Flora Thompson[†] described the wishing well as being, in 1898, 'a deep sandy basin fed by a spring of crystal clear water which gushed from the bank above' and said that it had dozens of pins at the bottom which had been dropped in it for luck. When she returned in the 1920s the water 'fell in a thin trickle from a lead pipe, the sandy basin having been filled in.' Today, although there is no longer a sandy basin, a new well invites the passer-by to throw in a coin for the benefit of The National Trust – and, of course, to make a wish.

10 Carry on down the path, turn left to cross the stream by the footbridge, and follow the bridle path to the right and up a sunken track. (If muddy, you may wish to take the alternative but steeper route on higher ground). At the crest of the hill keep following this track down and then steeply up the other side of a valley with the fence of Downlands Estate to your right. In about half a mile, after passing an area used as a car park, the track becomes a paved road.

To your left is the site of one of several Canadian camps from WW2 located on the commons here. Only the concrete tracks now remain.

11 After about half a mile, turn right down another paved road (Rectory Lane) and past the main entrance to *Downlands*. The road soon becomes one of the typical 'sunken lanes' of the region before emerging in Bramshott village. The road bears to the left arriving at a green triangle in the centre of the village. Take the right fork, cross over the road and enter the churchyard by the lych gate.

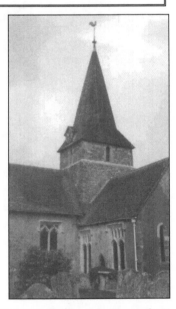

12 The church of St Mary, Bramshott ('only five years younger than the Magna Carta') is worth a visit. Follow the path through the churchyard to the right, then turn left past the rows of graves of 317 Canadian soldiers who died in the military hospital on Bramshott Common during the First World War – many from the influenza epidemic in late 1918 rather than from enemy action.

St Mary's Church, Bramshott

On the other side of the churchyard wall, to your left, note the rear of *Bramshott Manor* which is said to be one of the oldest continually inhabited houses in Hampshire, dating as it does from the year 1220.

[†] *Heatherley* by Flora Thompson

Follow the path out of the back of the churchyard – it is known locally as 'The Hanger' – under the A3 Liphook bypass bridge to meet the old London Road.

13 Turn right towards the bridge taking the road over the river. From here, follow the pavement along the road into Liphook.

> Note to the right of the road bridge an old aqueduct over the river, part of a large network of irrigation sluices and channels which stretched for miles along the valley. These were designed to obtain a second annual harvest of animal fodder by flooding the riverside meadows at intervals.

14 As you near the centre of Liphook, note the plaque on a house to the left commemorating Flora Thompson, author of 'Lark Rise to Candleford' – she was the postmaster's wife here for 12 years. Turn left at the second mini-roundabout in the town centre, opposite *The Royal Anchor*, then right at the next. Follow the road back to the station, keeping right where the road swings left to Sainsbury's and eventually turning right just before the road goes over the railway bridge. Turn left at the *Railway Arms* for the station entrance.

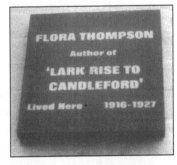

Plaque to Flora Thompson in London Road, Liphook

> Flora Thompson, author of *Lark Rise to Candleford*, achieved fame late in life. During her 12 years in Liphook in the 1920s she wrote much but her talent was unrecognised at this stage. Her nature notes, *The Peverel Papers*, written at this time have now been published in full and show some of the thoughts, places and characters she was to include in her more famous work more than a decade later.
>
> Another of her lesser-known works, *Heatherley*, written as a sequel to *Lark Rise to Candleford*, tells of her life in nearby Grayshott at the end of the 19th century.

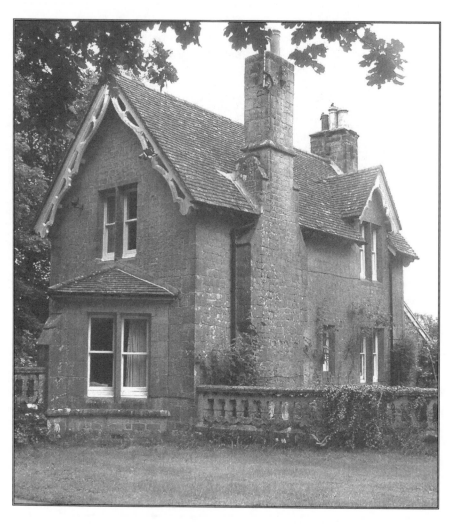

Lodge house at Foley Manor

Circular Walk 9 – Liphook & Griggs Green

Visiting: The Black Fox, Langley, Weavers Down,
Griggs Green and Foley Manor
Distance approximately 7½ miles/12km

The walk starts and ends at Liphook Station, passing several pubs

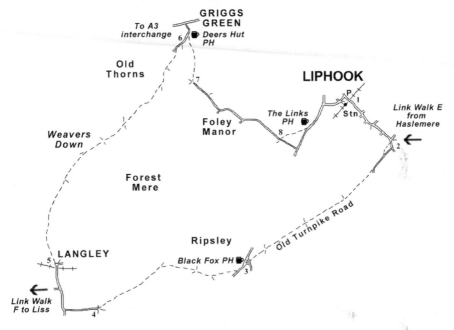

1   Turn right out of the station and into the car park. Take the steps up to the road bridge, and cross the railway line. Follow the road, crossing to use the pavements as necessary. Just past the 'Welcome to West Sussex' sign, turn right down a path which soon merges with a vehicular track. This is the route of an old turnpike road from London to Portsmouth.

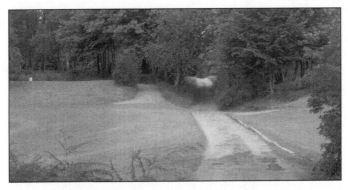

The old turnpike road going across the golf course

47

2 Follow the old turnpike which takes a fairly straight course for about a mile and a half, through woodland, past gated houses and across a golf course, before meeting the later Portsmouth Road opposite the *Black Fox Inn*.

3 Cross the road with care, and take a bridleway to the right just past the pub. Follow this through a gate and past Liphook cricket ground, taking the centre track where paths divide, then left where it meets a sunken track coming in from the right. After another gate, the bridleway meets a surfaced lane.

4 Go straight ahead along the surfaced lane to meet another lane at a T-junction. Turn right and pass Little Langley Farm. *Note: To follow Link Walk F to Liss and all points south, turn left down the lane just after Little Langley Farm.* To continue Circular Walk 9, keep straight ahead here to cross the railway line on a road bridge.

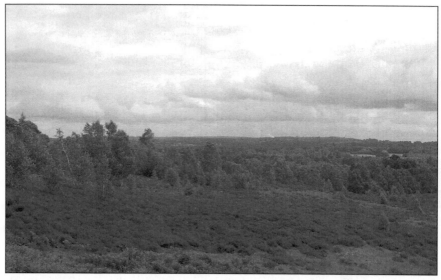

View from Weavers Down looking south-east

5 At a small grass triangle, bear slightly left then take the bridleway which diverges to the right by the gateway to a house. Follow this as it heads towards Weavers Down and its prominent aerial assembly in the distance. After a while it climbs to higher ground following the Hampshire/Sussex border, and there are views to the right. It passes another golf course to the left, then descends to Griggs Green and the welcome sight of the *Deers Hut* pub.

6 If you are not going into the pub, your route turns sharp right here – alternatively, coming out of the *Deers Hut*, turn left to follow the line of buildings. Follow the track past some houses, then continue on the bridleway as it passes through light woodland. It can be extremely muddy here. Shortly after a barn on the left, turn left onto a surfaced lane.

7   Follow the road through the Foley Manor estate with its ornamental ponds. Note the statue of Field Marshal Hugh Henry Rose, 1st Baron Strathnairn, GCSI KCB, 1801–1885 on horseback by the front drive to the manor house. This was first erected to his memory at Knightsbridge, and later moved to Foley.

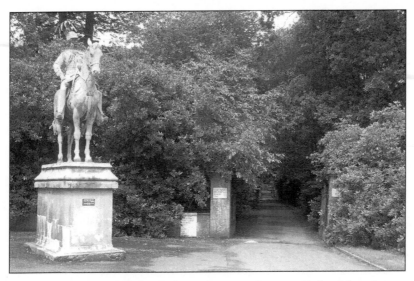

Statue of Field Marshal Hugh Henry Rose at Foley Manor

8   Just after the lodge house (photographed by Flora Thompson in her *Peverel Papers* of March 1922), take a bridleway to the left. This cuts though behind the golf course to arrive at a main road by *The Links* inn. Follow the road into Liphook, turning right along Station Road and past an arcade of shops to arrive back at the station.

Link Walk F – Liphook to Liss

Visiting: The Black Fox and Langley
Distance approximately 6 miles/9.5km

The walk starts at Liphook Station and ends at Liss Station

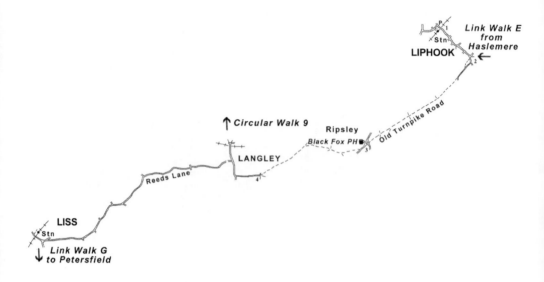

Start by following Circular Walk 9 from Liphook Station to Point 4 (see details earlier) where the bridleway meets a surfaced lane.

Continue to follow Circular Walk 9 straight ahead along the surfaced lane to meet another lane at a T-junction. Turn right and pass Little Langley Farm.

For **Link Walk F**, turn left down a lane shortly afterwards and follow the right of way marked for traffic along the lanes until arriving in Liss.

If continuing to Petersfield and all points south along **Link Walk G**, turn left at the mini-roundabout in the centre of Liss, otherwise turn right here to arrive at Liss station.

Circular Walk 10 – Liss & Hawkley

Visiting: *Liss Forest, Greatham, Hawkley and West Liss*
Distance approximately 9 miles/14.5km

The walk starts and ends at Liss Station;
refreshment at *The Hawkley Inn*

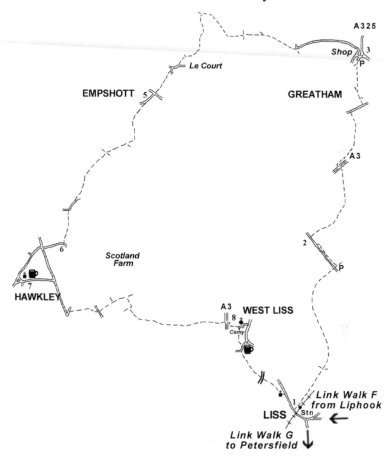

1 From the station forecourt, cross the level crossing and shortly turn right to follow the Liss Riverside Walk along an old railway track (the military railway to Longmoor and Bordon – note the old platform on the right – see next page) for just over a mile until it meets a road. Turn left along the road for about a third of a mile (there is a more interesting parallel track through woodland to the right for part of the way), passing the Greatham Treatment Works before turning right along a public bridleway.

2 Follow the bridleway which passes a pond on the left and crosses the A3 road on a footbridge after about half a mile, then turns right and passes through woodland to meet a road. Turn right here passing houses on the right, then at

the end of the houses turn left along a public footpath. Bear left where paths first divide, then follow the main path through plantations to arrive at a gravel parking area off a roundabout on the A325.

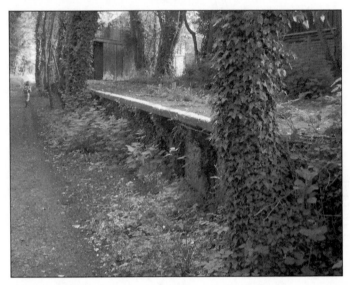

The old platform for the Longmoor Military Railway at Liss

The Longmoor Military Railway was part of the Army railway system which once ran from Bordon Camp via Longmoor Camp to Liss. Originally designed in 1903 to train soldiers at Longmoor on railway construction and operations, the extension to Liss was opened in 1933.

The system was closed in October 1969.

3   Turn left along Digby Way, the short connecting road to Greatham, then turn right past the shop and follow the road (Benhams Lane) as it bends left. Keep straight on to Benhams Farm. Here, as the road bears right, take the footpath straight ahead through a gate to the right of the farmhouse. Follow the right of way as best you can across a field, over a wooden bridge and across another field. Take the left fork where the way splits in the middle of this last field, though the path was not obvious at the time of writing, eventually going over a couple of stiles and onto a track. Turn left along the track and follow it across a field, leading to where a stile stands by a hedge. Turn right here and follow the hedge at the edge of the field as it rises towards a wood. There are good views to the right.

4   Go through a gap in the corner of the field and across a plank bridge, then along a narrow path bordered on the left by a high wire fence surrounding an orchard. Go into the orchard through a small wooden gate through the fence by a metal gate, and follow the track round the top of the orchard and past a dilapidated building, bearing right at a hedge, then going out of the orchard

through a wide metal gate on the left. Follow the track ahead which passes Le Court buildings on the left.

Le Court was the site of the first of the Cheshire homes, opened in 1948 as a residential home for disabled ex-servicemen. The home was closed down in 2002.

Pass though a barrier, then as the drive bears left take the footpath straight ahead going downhill across a field. Cross a stile and a plank bridge and go though some woodland to arrive at a road junction.

5　Cross the road with care and go along Church Lane straight ahead, soon taking a farm track going downhill to the left. Follow this – eventually it becomes less distinct, just some ruts (see below) crossing a field and rising to a gate.

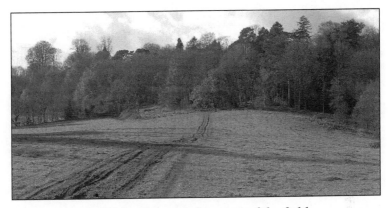

Head for the top left corner of the field

Turn left <u>in front of</u> this gate and follow the track to the top left corner of the field where it goes through another gate and becomes more prominent again, rising along the edge of a wood and eventually becoming a metalled lane. Shortly after this, take a footpath up a bank to the left and across fields to arrive at a road.

6　Turn right at the road, past a pond, to arrive at a T-junction. Turn right and left taking the road to Hawkley. In the village, turn left in front of the church and left again to arrive at the *Hawkley Inn*, which can be recommended for refreshment.

The Hangers Way, a 21-mile recreational path from the South Downs to Alton, passes through Hawkley. The 'hangers' are steep-sided wooded escarpments such as the one described by Gilbert White in his *Natural History of Selborne*.

7   Turn left out of the inn, following the road to a T-junction. Turn right and follow the road with care as it goes downhill and bears sharply left. Halfway down the next stretch, take a footpath up the bank to the right. Use this to cross a couple of fields and cut out a bend in the road. Rejoining the road, cross over and take a lane almost directly opposite. Follow this for a few hundred yards then take a footpath over a stile to the right. Follow this by a fence as it winds its way across streams and over stiles to emerge in a field. Turn left along the left side of the field to a stile and gate. Go through more fields with stile and gate options, finally joining a track which crosses the A3 again on a footbridge after about three-quarters of a mile in total.

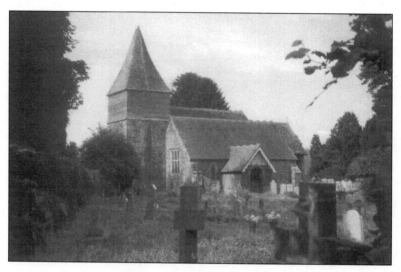

St Peter's Church, West Liss

8   After crossing the A3 the path bears right to enter a field. The diagonal path shown crossing the field on the map does not seem to exist, so turn left along the field edge to arrive at Liss Cemetery. Opposite is the old church of St Peter's, West Liss. Go through the cemetery and follow the footpath out at the other end. The path crosses a couple of roads before entering the churchyard of St Mary's, East Liss in about half a mile. The last section was once an old coaching road. Turn left in front of the vestry door and exit the churchyard by the main gate. Turn right here to follow the road back to Liss station.

Link Walk G – Liss to Petersfield

Distance approximately 4½ miles/7km

The walk starts at Liss Station and ends at Petersfield Station; refreshment at the *Harrow*, Steep

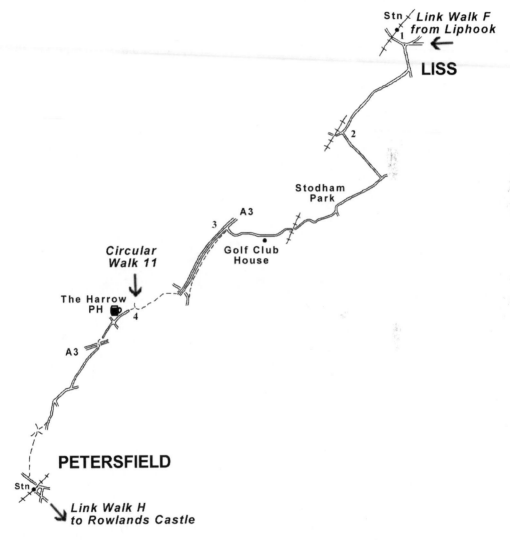

1 From Liss station, turn left past the shops and bear right at the mini-roundabout. In about 250yards, turn right along Andlers Ash Road and follow this for half a mile.

2 Just before the railway level crossing, turn left along Stodham Lane. Follow this as it rises gently, bearing right at a triangular junction at the top of the

hill. Bear right at Stodham Park and follow the lane across the river. Bear left in front of the gates to The Dragon House where the surfacing ends and cross the railway line at a pedestrian level crossing (taking normal precautions). Soon the lane becomes surfaced once more, and Petersfield Golf Club course is on both sides of you. Follow the lane to its junction with the dual carriageway of the A3.

3   Turn left along the cycle & footpath by the edge of the road, following it as it soon bears left and descends to a junction with a smaller road. Turn right along this road under the A3, then after the bridge take a track immediately to the left. Cross a stile by a metal gate and go up steps to the right. Follow the footpath round the edge of a field, then through woodland to emerge by some houses facing a stream.

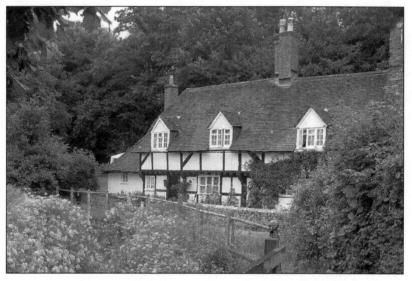

Houses by the stream near to The Harrow, Steep

4   Turn left to arrive shortly at *The Harrow Inn* (see p.59). From here follow Circular Walk 11 (from Point 9) to Petersfield Station.

Circular Walk 11 – Petersfield & Steep

Visiting: Steep, the 'Shoulder of Mutton' hill and 'The Harrow'
Distance approximately 6 miles/9.5km with one severe climb

**The walk starts and ends at Petersfield Station;
refreshment at *The Harrow Inn* after 4¾ miles**

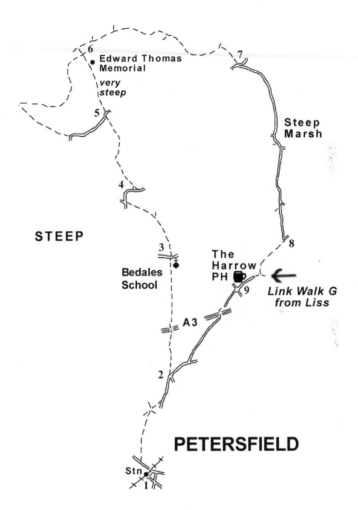

1   Turn left out of the station and cross the line at the level crossing (or foot-bridge). Follow the road for about 100 yards before taking a footpath to the right next to a car sales showroom. Look for small labels on lamp posts, etc, indicating the 'Hangers Way' – we will follow this to the Shoulder of Mutton Hill. Carry on along the path for just over 200 yards, crossing a track before descending to join a road. Follow the road to the left for a short distance to a bend.

2   Where the road bends to the right, take the path through a gate straight ahead. This crosses the A3 dual carriageway by a footbridge and, with Bedales School on the left, arrives at the side of All Saints' Church, Steep.

> Bedales was founded in 1893 by John Haden Badley as a liberal alternative to the authoritarian regimes customary in independent schools of the time. It has been coeducational since 1898 and claims many renowned ex-pupils.

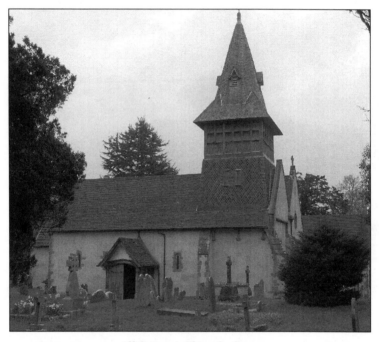

All Saints' Church, Steep

3   Cross the road, pass through a gate and go across a small playing field. The path continues through a wood and descends to a stile. From here the path skirts a field and it can get very muddy. Pass though an iron kissing-gate to a road. Turn right and follow the road downhill to a bend.

4   At the bend, take the footpath straight ahead past a waterfall. Turn left at the top, and follow the path past a series of lakes on the left, eventually arriving at a road.

5   Here you have a choice of routes. The official Hangers Way turns left and follows a fairly lengthy and muddy diversion to the top of Shoulder of Mutton Hill avoiding a very steep climb. Unless you find the climb impossible, we recommend instead that you turn right and immediately left to follow a path and steps straight up the side of the 'Shoulder of Mutton' hill.

6   After passing the Edward Thomas memorial stone, stopping to admire the view behind you and getting your breath back, carry straight on, soon to meet a bridleway. Turn right here along an un-surfaced lane, following the Hangers Way sign. Shortly the Hangers Way leaves us to the left across a stile – keep straight ahead along the lane, and straight ahead again when another lane goes off to the left. The lane descends gently along a ridge with a wooded 'hanger' to the right, then more steeply. Towards the bottom of the steep section, look for a stile and footpath to the right. This takes you through an avenue of trees and across a field to a stile by road.

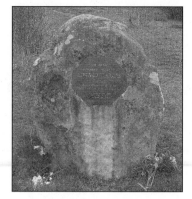

Edward Thomas memorial stone on the 'Shoulder of Mutton' hill

7   Turn right along the road, then almost immediately sharp left at a junction. Follow the road downhill for about half a mile to the hamlet of Steep Marsh. Bear right at a road junction here (signposted Sheet & Petersfield) and in another 500 yards or so keep straight ahead where the major road bears left. Follow this past roadside buildings on the right and down to a bend. Take the bridleway to the right.

8   Follow the bridleway as it goes along the left-hand shoulder of an old sunken lane, now next to impassable, arriving at lovely old half-timbered houses by a stream. Continue past the houses and over a bridge. The path becomes a metalled lane. Follow this uphill to arrive at *The Harrow Inn*, a very suitable place to take on refreshment (but note, children not allowed inside).

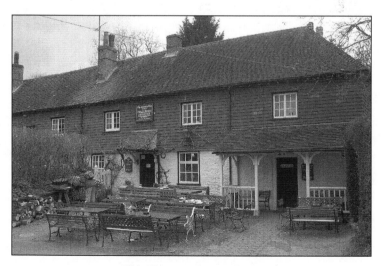

The Harrow Inn at Steep

9 Leaving the Harrow Inn, go straight ahead at the crossroads and along a lane which has now been cut in two by the A3 dual carriageway. Cross this by another footbridge, and continue along the lane which starts again on the other side, eventually arriving at Point 2 of the outward journey. Retrace your steps from here to Petersfield station, carrying on along the road for a couple of hundred yards before taking a path bearing uphill to the right. After crossing another track bear left where the path splits. This passes behind house gardens and descends to a road. Turn left here for the station.

Edward Thomas (1878–1917), poet and journalist, lived in Steep when he enlisted into the Army in 1915. He was killed in action at Arras.

On 6th August 1853, John Bonham-Carter of Petersfield started the excavation of Buriton Tunnel for the new railway line. According to reports, 'a handsome mahogany barrow was rapidly filled with earth – and with bouquets of flowers thrown in by the ladies present'.

Trains did not begin to run until January 1859, and even then a dispute between railway companies held up full use of the line through to Portsmouth until 8th May.

We join the South Downs Way for part of Walk 12, from Butser Hill through Queen Elizabeth Country Park – a long-distance footpath and bridleway stretching for about 100 miles between Winchester and Eastbourne.

Queen Elizabeth Country Park contains some 20 miles of trails for walkers, cyclists and horse riders. Refreshments are available in its Coach-house café.

Buriton, the original mother-village of Petersfield, has two good pubs and a large village duck pond in front of the church.

Circular Walk 12 – Petersfield, Butser & Buriton

Visiting: Butser Hill, Queen Elizabeth Country Park and Buriton
Distance approximately 11 miles/17.5km with gradients

**The walk starts and ends at Petersfield Station;
refreshment at Queen Elizabeth Country Park and Buriton**

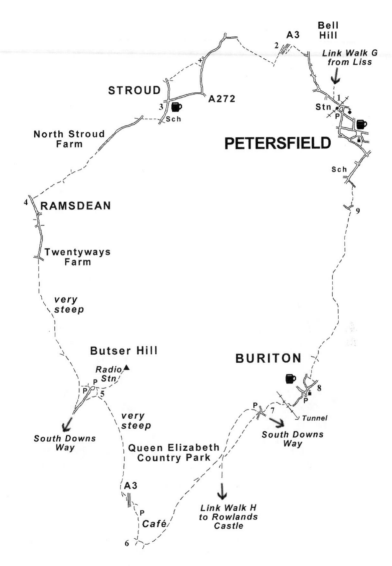

1   Turn left out of the station main entrance and cross the line at the level crossing (or footbridge). Follow the road, bearing right at a roundabout to go up Bell Hill. Near the top of the hill, turn left just before a post box and follow a track which becomes a public footpath at its end. Go over the stile

and shortly turn right through a kissing gate and cross the A3 on a pedestrian footbridge.

2   Turn left off the bridge, following the footpath down the side of a field and over another two stiles. Turn right at the second stile, and follow the footpath across fields and stiles to arrive at the end of a lane by Mellstock Farm. Go down this to its T-junction with a road. Turn left along the road, soon passing the diminutive Stroud Church. Shortly after this, take a footpath between hedges to the right. (This can get overgrown in the growing season – if it looks impassable, keep to the road and turn right at its junction with the A272 to rejoin our route). The footpath opens out to cross fields and stiles and arrives at the track to Rothercombe Farm. Turn left here to meet the A272 in Stroud, almost opposite the *Seven Stars* pub.

3   Cross the road with care and take the lane (Ramsdean Road) directly opposite. Just past the village school, take a footpath to the right. Pass through several kissing gates to arrive at a lane. Turn left and follow this lane (which becomes unsurfaced after North Stroud Farm) for a mile to Ramsdean.

4   Turn left along the road through Ramsdean and follow it for nearly half a mile to a T-junction at Twentyways Farm. There are in fact only four ways here – go straight ahead through a metal gate on a by-way track and follow it for over a mile as it rises, at one point rather steeply, towards Butser Hill.

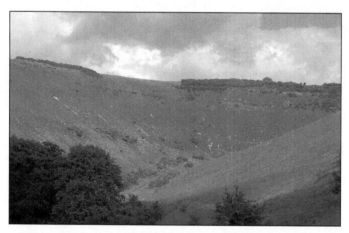

View of Grandfather's Bottom on the climb to Butser Hill

Butser Hill may be accessed by way of an unmarked footpath giving a scrambling climb to the left before the track arrives at a road – if you miss it, turn sharp left at the road instead (signposted South Downs Way) and follow it to the car park. At 270 metres (886 feet) Butser Hill is the highest point in Hampshire. If you wish to reach the summit, follow the tracks past the radio mast to the triangulation point. The hill has a rather flat top and you have to walk a fair distance to find the edges and get the best views.

5 From the car park, follow signs for the South Downs Way which descends steeply down the south side of the hill before going under the A3 to arrive at the buildings of the Queen Elizabeth Country Park. There is a restaurant and a souvenir shop here.

6 Continue along the South Downs Way or take the Hangers Way – both go in the same direction but by slightly different routes, eventually joining at Halls Hill car park.

7 Cross straight over the road and take the bridleway waymarked Hangers Way which descends through old chalk pit workings and under a railway bridge to arrive at Buriton pond and its friendly ducks. There are two excellent pubs nearby, up the road to the left.

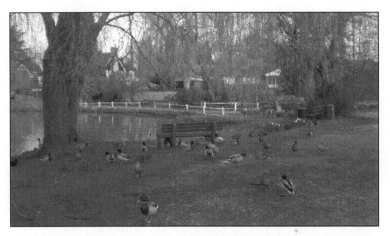

Be prepared to share your lunch at Buriton pond!

8 To continue the walk, follow the Hangers Way signs, following the road as it bends to the left past the pond then taking a left turn up a residential road and turning right at the 'Hop Loft' house. Soon take a gate to the left to follow a path along the edge of a steep-sided grassy valley. This path continues over stiles and through fields, very muddy in places, for a mile and a half to the outskirts of Petersfield.

9 Go into a mobile home estate, follow signs to the right to 'Office' then, just before the office building, turn left over a plank bridge and through a weighted wicket gate. Carry on along the path across a field and down a drive to arrive at a main road opposite The Petersfield School entrance. Turn right and go along the pavement into Petersfield town. All the usual shops and refreshment houses await you before you head back to the station.

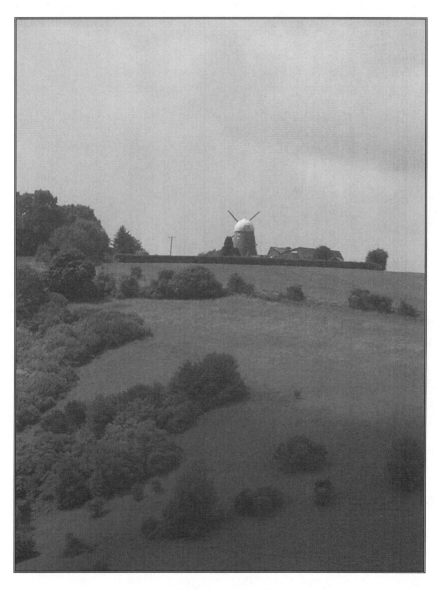

Chalton windmill

Link Walk H – Petersfield to Rowlands Castle

Visiting: Buriton, Chalton and Finchdean
Distance approximately 7 miles/11km

The walk starts at Petersfield Station and ends at Rowlands Castle Station; refreshment at the *Red Lion*, Chalton or *The George*, Finchdean

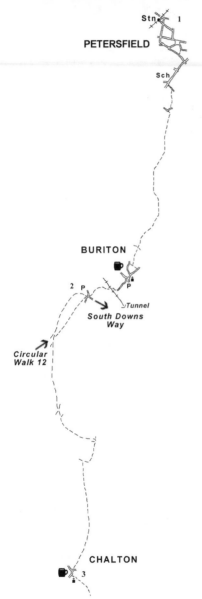

1 From Petersfield station, follow the Hangers Way (Circular Walk 12 in a reverse direction) through Buriton, past the duck pond and up the hill to a road junction by Halls Hill car park.

2 Follow the sign for the Hangers Way over the stile to the left of the car park entrance, taking the path through fields then rising through woodland to meet to a T-junction with a forest track. Turn left and follow this track (marked with a red footprint sign) continuing straight ahead in about three-quarters of a mile where it crosses another track. Here it joins the Staunton Way (waymarked with the picture of a roe deer and a green arrow) which you follow for about a mile and a half, turning left over a stile and crossing open fields to Chalton. Note the windmill on the brow of a hill to your right as you cross the fields. On arriving in Chalton, the *Red Lion* is straight ahead of you – supposedly the oldest pub in Hampshire.

3 Enter the churchyard opposite the *Red Lion* through a lych gate and continue following the Staunton Way which now, while still deep in Hampshire, shares its route to Rowlands Castle with the Sussex Border Path.

65

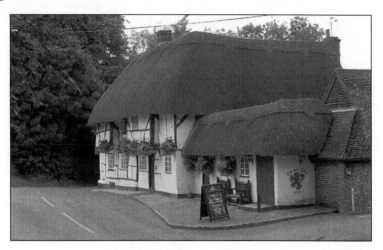

The Red Lion at Chalton

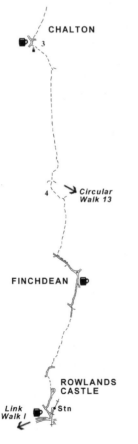

Go through a kissing gate and cross a couple of stiles before taking the right-most of three dividing tracks. Follow this uphill and past a tumulus – there are views to right and left – note Idsworth Church in a field beyond the railway line to the left. After passing under pylons the track changes sides of a fence by going across a stile, then goes round a copse to arrive at a cross-roads of paths.

4 For Circular Walk 13, turn left – to continue this link walk to Rowlands Castle carry straight on and round the edge of a field, turning right at the end. *From here you follow Circular Walk 13 in a reverse direction.* After joining a road, pass through the village of Finchdean – turn right in the middle of the village, pass *The George* then take a road uphill to the right, bearing left along a track where the road turns right. The way soon passes a gate and heads across an open field to arrive at Rowlands Castle.

The railway station is well signposted, but if you wish to continue your walk to Havant, carry on through the village – see Link Walk I.

Circular Walk 13 – Rowlands Castle & West Marden

Visiting: Finchdean, Idsworth Church, West Marden, Stansted Park
Distance approximately 8¾ miles/14km

**The walk starts and ends at Rowlands Castle Station;
refreshment at the *Victoria Inn*, West Marden**

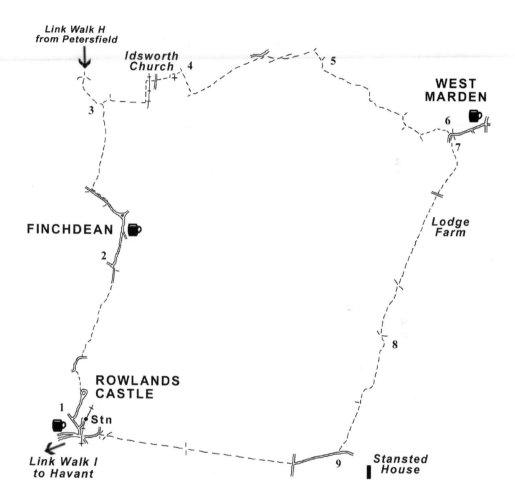

1 Turn left out of the station and walk down the approach road. Turn right along the road at the bottom, and shortly right again along Uplands Road. Towards the end of this road, where it loops round a grassed area, take a footpath between houses on the left. Follow this as it becomes a track and meets a lane (Wellsworth Lane). Turn right along the lane, passing a house on the left before following the Sussex Border Path sign to the left at a junction. Once an old hedged track, this is now an open path across a large hedgeless field, regaining its original form only just before joining a road.

2 Turn right down the road and into the village of Finchdean. Turn left in the centre of the village, along the road opposite *The George Inn*. Where Ashcroft Lane comes in on the right, look for a gap in the hedge on the right. Go through the gap and follow the waymarked Sussex Border Path along the bottom edge of the field and then up its left hand side. There are good views to the right and bluebell woods in season to the left as the path climbs the hill.

3 At the top of the hill, just after passing through a narrow band of trees, take a track to the right which drops in a straight line to the valley below. There is a good 'aerial' view of Idsworth church from here. You will be there soon.

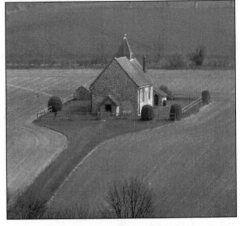

At the bottom, turn left for a few yards, then right under the railway to meet a road. *Note: after wet weather the passage under the railway can be flooded.* Turn left along the road, then almost immediately right along a path leading up through a field to the church.

'Aerial' view of Idsworth church viewed from the opposite hill

> St Hubert's Church, Idsworth, also called "The Little Church in a Field" for obvious reasons, contains wall paintings said to be "the oldest in Christendom," dated c.1330. It is usually open, and well worth a visit.

4 Passing the left side of the church, go across the field to a stile, turn right along a hedge, and bear left at the bottom of the field. Continue along the field edge, crossing another stile before taking a footpath to the right diagonally up the side of a hill. The path enters woodland through a kissing gate and rises up a short flight of steps to join a larger track. Turn left, still going uphill. In about fifty yards take a public footpath leading up another flight of steps to the right – follow the path uphill through woodland to a T-junction with a bridleway.

5 Turn right and proceed along a farm track which winds between hedges. Keep right at the first junction, and after about three-quarters of a mile in total take a footpath which drops to the left. Towards the bottom it has been diverted in a series of landscaped bends to avoid the grounds of West Marden Hall. After this it meets a road.

6 Turn left towards the village of West Marden. Almost immediately, our path home goes off to the right – but if you are in need of sustenance, carry on a short way down the road to find the *Victoria Inn* on the left, returning here afterwards.

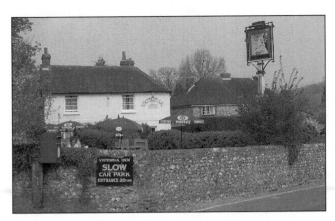

The Victoria Inn at West Marden

7   Take the right-most of the two footpaths over the stile opposite West Marden Hall. Go up the hill across the field and over the stile at the top. Turn left and follow the narrow path between fence and woodland uphill, eventually coming out onto an open field. Looking behind you, you can see Uppark House in the distance across a valley. Continue across the field beside a hedge, over a lane and through a farm, then across another open field and into woodland. Follow the bridleway through the woods (it can be muddy) to emerge at the edge of a field with a distant view of the sea.

8   Continue down the bridleway through the edge of a wood to meet a surfaced drive at a wooden gate.

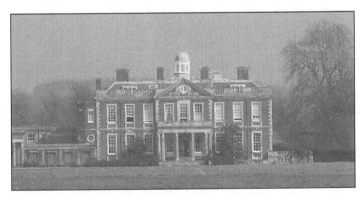

Stansted House from The Avenue

9   Turn right along the drive and through the exit gates of Stansted Park. Cross straight over a road and through a small metal gate opposite onto The Avenue – an impressively wide grassy 'ride' over a mile long from Stansted House to Rowlands Castle. At the end, a path leads through trees and down to a road. Turn left here and go under a railway bridge, then right to return to the station.

Link Walk I – Rowlands Castle to Havant

Distance approximately 3¾ miles/6km

The walk starts at Rowlands Castle Station and ends at Havant station; refreshment at Rowlands Castle and Havant

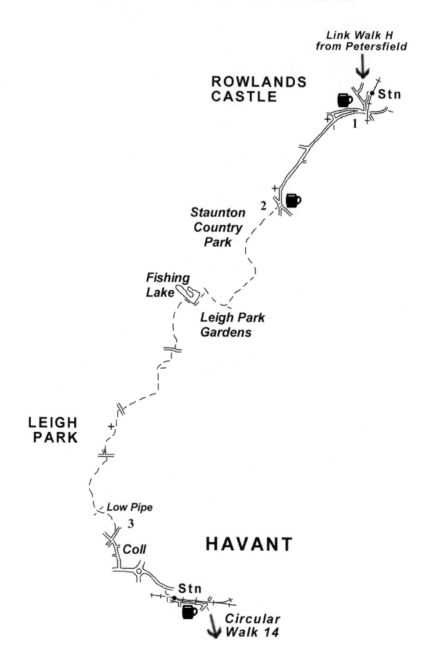

1 From Rowlands Castle station road, turn left then right, away from the bridge, and follow the pavement along the road on the left side of the green. Continue along this road (Redhill Road) to a roundabout. Cross the road with care, turn left then shortly take a track to the right, opposite a pub. Pass through a gate into Staunton Country Park.

2 Follow the Staunton Way through the park by Leigh Park Gardens, past the fishing lake and continue south alongside the stream which issues from the lake.

This should be waymarked as the Staunton Way, but at the time of writing (October 2008) there were no signs in evidence. The route from the pond to the first road is particularly boggy and obscure and seems to require crossing an open ditch at one point! After that, take the metal kissing gate opposite and follow the path through woodland, then along the stream edge on one side or the other as best you can, sometimes through housing estates.

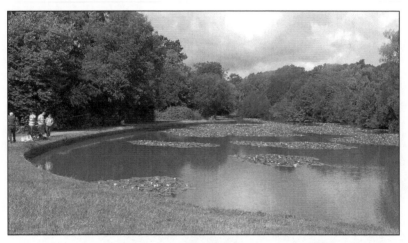

The fishing lake in Staunton Country Park

3 Shortly after passing under a large pipe (mind your head!) the path joins a road (Stockheath Lane) at a sign saying "Hermitage Stream, Hermit's Lea". At a T-junction, turn left onto Barncroft Way and go past the entrance to Havant College. Turn left at the next T-junction along New Road. At the large roundabout go straight ahead into Elmleigh Road. Just past the Magistrate's Court, turn right and across a footbridge over the railway line to the main entrance of the station.

To continue to Hayling Island and Portsmouth, follow Circular Walk 14.

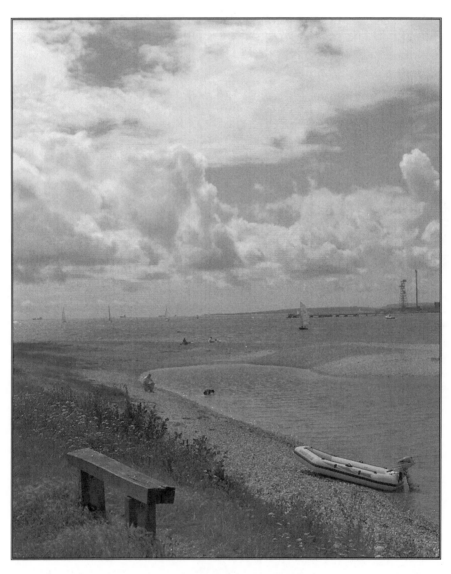

West coast at Hayling Island

Circular Walk 14 – Havant & Hayling Island

Visiting: Langstone, Hayling Billy coastal path, Stoke village, Northney
Distance approximately 8½ miles/13.5km

**The walk starts and ends at Havant Station; refreshment at
the *Royal Oak* and *Ship Inn*, Langstone and the *Yew Tree*, Stoke**

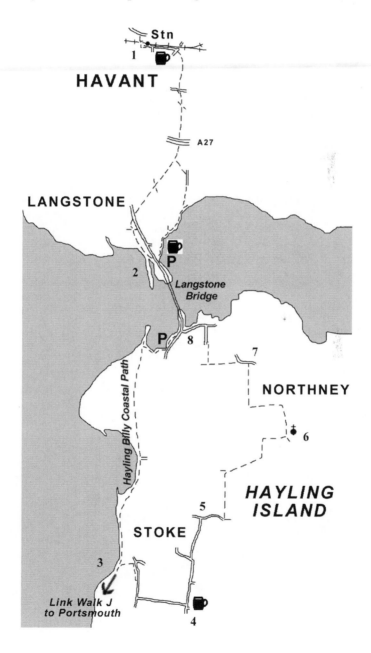

1   From the main (southern) entrance to Havant station, turn left through the car park. Cross the road at the end, going through old level crossing gates (this is the old track of the Hayling Billy line). Follow the course of the old line under two road bridges. Shortly after the second (and larger) bridge, note a footpath to the left across a bridge over a stream. Take this and follow the footpath past Wade Court to the coast. Turn right here and follow the coastal path, passing in front of the *Royal Oak* pub before arriving at the *Ship Inn* by Langstone Bridge. (Note that very high tides may make this route impassable in places).

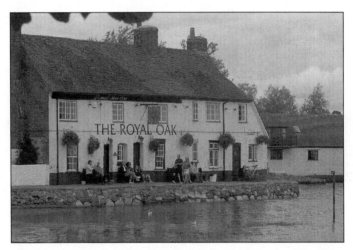

The Royal Oak at Langstone

2   Turn left and cross Langstone Bridge to the island. Cut right at the end of the bridge along a track leading to the Hayling Billy Coastal Path. Follow this down the west coast of the island for a mile and a half. There are interesting detours to be made to the right around the old oyster beds if you wish, and views over to Portsmouth.

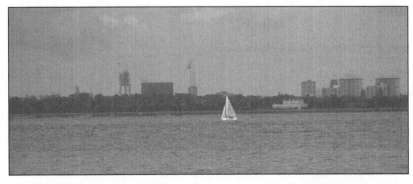

View to the Spinnaker Tower from Hayling Island

If you are walking all the way to Portsmouth (see Link Walk J), continue south along the coastal path and take the foot ferry across to Portsea Island.

3 To return to Havant, turn left in front of a large brick pill-box to take a path inland. Where this meets a road, turn right along a parallel bridleway, then join the road briefly (take care here) before taking Daw Lane to the left. Follow Daw Lane to its junction with the main Havant Road.

4 Turn left at Havant Road along a pavement through the village. The *Yew Tree* across the road is a possible refreshment stop. There are also shops here. Continue through the village and when the road bends left, turn right along Castlemans Lane. (Take great care here – the traffic can be unremitting – we suggest you walk past the bend and cross at the bus stop).

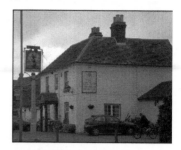

The Yew Tree Inn

5 At the end of the lane by Middlestoke Farm-house turn right along a farm track, pass some farm buildings and follow the track as it bends left. Continue along the track as it bends right and left across open fields. As it approaches houses, take a footpath left through a wooden barrier and into the churchyard of St Peter's Church, which dates from 1140.

6 Follow the footpath across the churchyard then along the edge of a field, turning left then right to follow the boundary, arriving eventually at a road.

7 Turn left along the road, then carry straight on along a drive where the road bears right. Pass a house and turn right along a field edge just before a stile. The path passes through the hedge and to a drive leading to the coastal road.

The Ordnance Survey map shows a bridleway leading straight ahead across the estuary at this point – it is not recommended!

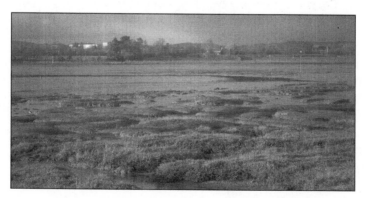

Start of the track across the estuary at low tide

8 Turn left then right to regain the mainland across Langstone Bridge. To return to Havant from there you may retrace your outward path or, for variety, follow the disused Hayling Billy railway track opposite the *Ship Inn*.

Link Walk J – Havant to Portsmouth Harbour

Visiting: Langstone, Hayling Billy coastal path, Hayling Island West Town,
Fort Cumberland, Eastney, Southsea
Distance approximately 14 miles/22.5km

The walk starts at Havant Station and ends at Portsmouth Harbour station; refreshment at *The Ferry Boat Inn* and locations in Southsea and Portsmouth

Follow Circular Walk 14 from Havant station to point 3, then continue south along the Hayling Billy Coastal Path. When it terminates at the old station, carry straight on along Staunton Road and turn right at the end along Sea Front. This becomes Ferry Road and leads to the foot ferry which crosses to Portsea Island. *The Ferry Boat Inn* offers refreshment here.

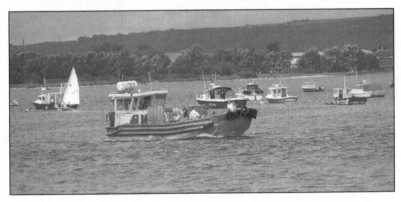

The foot ferry between Hayling Island and Portsea Island
Check ferry times and fares at www.langstoneharbour.org.uk/harbour/ferry.htm
Tel: 023 9248 2868

From the ferry landing, take the road past Fort Cumberland to the start of the Esplanade which runs all the way along the coast to Southsea. Follow this, picking up the Millennium walkway (and Walk 15) after you pass Clarence Pier and its fun fair, arriving eventually at Portsmouth Harbour station.

See Walk 15 for details of interest between Clarence Pier and Portsmouth Harbour station.

Circular Walk 15 – Portsmouth Harbour & Southsea

Visiting: Portsmouth & Southsea historic seafronts
Distance approximately 3 miles/5km

The walk starts and ends at Portsmouth Harbour Station; refreshment available at many locations on this route!

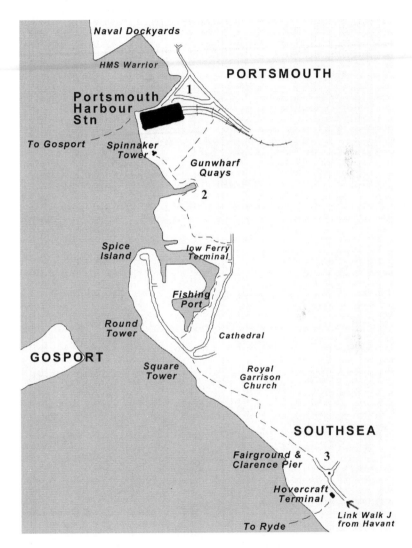

1   From the station entrance, turn right and follow the pavement round to a pedestrian underpass under the railway line through to Gunwharf Quays. Take this and walk through the shopping centre to the sea. To your right is the Spinnaker Tower. Turn left to follow the Millennium walkway (see brick pattern inset into pavement, similar to that shown on p.80).

2   The walkway crosses a bridge, traverses the vehicle-marshalling area for the Isle of Wight Ferries (care needed here), and passes the fishing port then loops round 'Spice Island' and curls back on itself before meandering through the old fortifications and heading for Southsea.

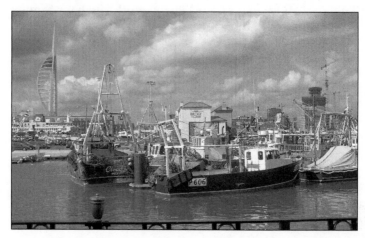

View across the fishing port at Portsmouth from the Millennium walkway, with the Isle of Wight ferry terminal and Spinnaker Tower in the background

Spice Island is a popular place to sit and watch the ships entering and leaving Portsmouth Harbour, with or without refreshment from the hostelries there!

There are plenty of interpretation boards along the route to tell you the history of the locations you pass.

3   The official Millennium walkway ends just before you arrive at Clarence Pier with its funfair. Walk through this to arrive at the hovercraft port.

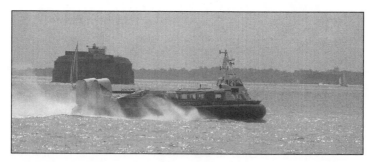

A hovercraft on its way from Southsea to the Isle of Wight

You may extend this walk along the esplanade to visit Southsea Castle and other attractions as you wish before retracing your steps. Alternatively, why not take advantage of the Hoverport to visit the Isle of Wight?

Circular Walk 15 – Optional extension to the Isle of Wight

The hovercraft takes you across the water to Ryde in 10 minutes. Check times and fares at **www.hovertravel.co.uk**

Once there you have a number of options:—

- Return to Southsea esplanade by hovercraft
- Return direct to Portsmouth Harbour station by high speed FastCat catamaran – see **www.wightlink.co.uk** for details
- Walk along the Coastal Path to Fishbourne (3 miles) via Quarr Abbey to catch the conventional ferry back to Portsmouth – see **www.wightlink.co.uk** for details

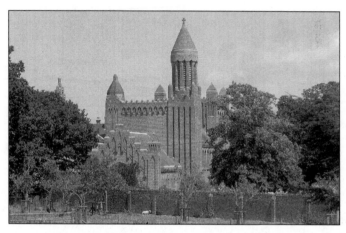

Quarr Abbey near Fishbourne, IoW

- Take the train from Ryde to Wootton (electric to Smallbrook Junction and steam to Wootton) and walk (about 2 miles) to the Fishbourne ferry from there, or take the return journey on the train back to Ryde.
  See details at **www.island-line.co.uk** and **www.iwsteamrailway.co.uk**

Note that the steam railway is seasonal and when it runs there are only about three return journeys per day between Smallbrook and Wootton.

Circular Walk 16 – Portsmouth Harbour & Gosport

Visiting: Submarine Museum, Fort Gilkicker, Stokes Bay, Central Gosport
Distance approximately 5 miles/8km

The walk starts and ends at Portsmouth Harbour Station;
refreshments available in Gosport

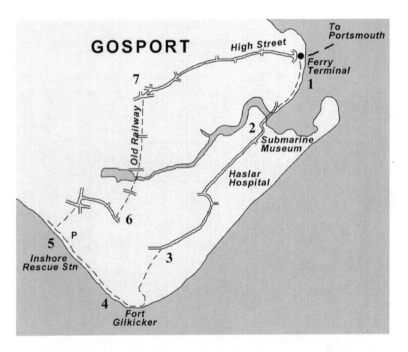

1   Take the foot-passenger ferry to Gosport from Portsmouth Harbour station.
From the landing jetty, turn left to follow the bricks of the Millennium Walk
along a walkway above Haslar Marina.

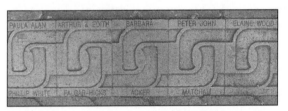

Sponsored bricks show the Millennium Walk at Gosport

After crossing a small footbridge it joins a road to pass over a larger one-way
traffic bridge controlled by lights. From the bridge there is a view to the left
of *HMS Alliance*, a hunter-killer post-war submarine now raised up out of the
water on stilts as part of the Royal Navy Submarine Museum.

80

2 Follow the road as it bears left then right to pass the Museum entrance. The Millennium bricks in the pavement stop here. Continue along a half-mile straight stretch of road between high brick walls. On the left is the Haslar Military Hospital. Turn left at the road junction to follow Clayhall Road for another half mile.

3 Just before the road narrows, take a track to the left (waymarked 'Solent Way') across a golf course towards Fort Gilkicker. This is one of a series of forts built in the 1860s as part of a ring of defences around Portsmouth. Follow a path which leads to the left of the fort, then turn right to walk along the shingle beach. The Isle of Wight car ferries from Portsmouth pass close to the shore here.

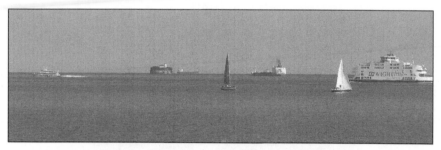

Isle of Wight ferry and other traffic at sea off Gilkicker Point

4 Continue along the beach or one of the parallel paths inland to arrive at the Stokes Bay Inshore Rescue station. There is a car park here and public conveniences. Note the view of Fawley oil refinery in the distance ahead.

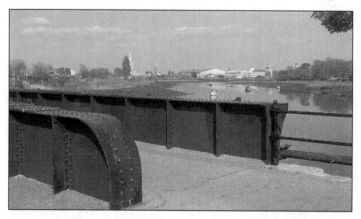

Old railway bridge now taking the cycle track

5 Turn right, either along the car park access road or across the playing fields, to arrive at the road again. Cross this near to a mini-roundabout and go along Anglesey Road opposite for a short distance, then right into Crescent Road.

Follow the road past ornamental gardens on the right and the Anglesey Hotel on the left, and turn left soon afterwards along a cycle/pedestrian track which follows the course of the old railway line. (This was originally built to take Queen Victoria to Stokes Bay where she caught a ferry to reach her Osborne House retreat on the Isle of Wight).

6 Follow the track. It crosses a number of roads and a couple of bridges arriving after about three-quarters of a mile at a main road. Cross this with care, taking a path to the road opposite which leads diagonally through the car park of the *White Hart* pub to another main road. Turn right here heading down Stoke Road for the centre of Gosport.

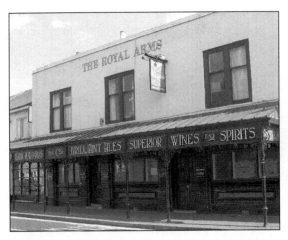

Elegant porch on The Royal Arms in central Gosport

7 Carry straight on for about a mile through the shopping centre of Gosport to return to the ferry terminal for Portsmouth Harbour station.

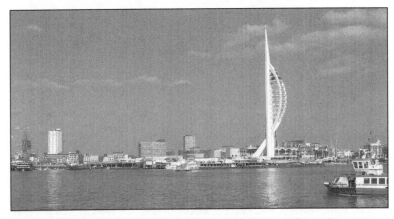

View of Portsmouth and the Spinnaker Tower from Gosport

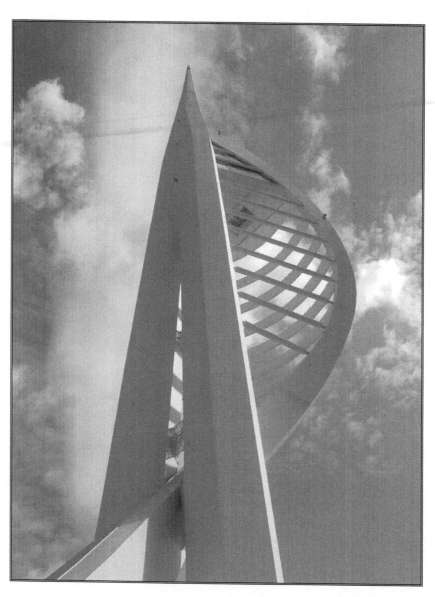

Destination mark: the Spinnaker at Portsmouth Harbour

Other local walks:—

Walks Around Headley ... and over the borders

A dozen circular walks starting from Headley.

ISBN 978-1-873855-49-2 with notes, illustrations and maps.

Walks Through History ... at the West of the Weald

A dozen circular walks with a historical theme.

ISBN 978-1-873855-51-5 with notes, illustrations and maps.

Walks Around Liphook

Booklet describing 20 circular walks in and around Liphook. *Bramshott & Liphook Preservation Society, 12 London Road, Liphook, Hants GU30 7AN.*

Other books of local interest:—

Heatherley – by Flora Thompson – *her sequel to the 'Lark Rise' trilogy*

The book which Flora Thompson wrote about her time in Grayshott – the 'missing' fourth part of her *Lark Rise to Candleford* collection.

ISBN 978-1-873855-29-4 September 1998, notes, illustrations and maps.

The Peverel Papers – by Flora Thompson – *her Nature Notes written in Liphook, 1921–1927.* Full and unabridged version

ISBN 978-1-873855-57-7 Published May 2008, notes, illustrations and maps.

On the Trail of Flora Thompson – from Grayshott to Griggs Green

Discovering the true life of Flora Thompson as she describes it in *Heatherley*.

ISBN 978-1-873855-24-9 First published May 1997, updated 2005.

Shottermill – its Farms, Families and Mills by Greta Turner

A history of Shottermill and the area around – where the counties of Hampshire, Surrey and Sussex meet. *Two volumes.*

ISBNs 978-1-873855-39-3 & 978-1-873855-40-9 Published 2004/2005.

The Hilltop Writers – a Victorian Colony among the Surrey Hills, by W.R. (Bob) Trotter

Rich in detail yet thoroughly readable, this book tells of sixty-six writers including Tennyson, Conan Doyle and Bernard Shaw who chose to work among the hills around Haslemere and Hindhead in the last decades of the 19th century.

ISBN 978-1-873855-31-7 Illustrated version, published March 2003.

John Owen Smith, publisher — www.johnowensmith.co.uk